Evaluating Clinical and Public Health Interventions

Evaluating clinical and public health interventions

A practical guide to study design and statistics

Mitchell H. Katz, MD

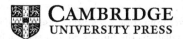
CAMBRIDGE
UNIVERSITY PRESS

CAMBRIDGE UNIVERSITY PRESS
Cambridge, New York, Melbourne, Madrid, Cape Town,
Singapore, São Paulo, Delhi, Mexico City

Cambridge University Press
The Edinburgh Building, Cambridge CB2 8RU, UK

Published in the United States of America by Cambridge University Press, New York

www.cambridge.org
Information on this title: www.cambridge.org/9780521735599

First published 2010

A catalogue record for this publication is available from the British Library

Library of Congress Cataloguing in Publication Data
Katz, Mitchell H.
    Evaluating clinical and public health interventions : a practical guide to study design and statistics /
Mitchell H. Katz.
       p. ; cm.
    Includes bibliographical references and index.
    ISBN 978-0-521-51488-0 (hardback) – ISBN 978-0-521-73559-9 (pbk.)
    1. Medical care–Evaluation–Methodology.   I. Title.
    [DNLM: 1. Evaluation Studies as Topic.   2. Research Design.   3. Statistics as Topic–methods.
    W 20.5 K215e 2010]
    RA399.A1K385 2010
    362.1068–dc22   2009054009

ISBN 978-0-521-51488-0 Hardback
ISBN 978-0-521-73559-9 Paperback

To Igael Gurin-Malous, with love

Contents

Preface

My experience as a public health director has taught me that solving complex health problems requires identifying useful interventions. This book is my intervention to make it easier (and more fun) to conduct intervention studies.[1]

Many different types of interventions can improve health and health care, including drugs and medical devices, laws and changes in medical and organizational practices. To enable you to evaluate a wide range of interventions, this book explains the advantages and disadvantages of many different approaches: randomized and nonrandomized studies; prospective and retrospective studies; planned clinical trials and observational studies (e.g., studies using administrative databases, disease registries); evaluations of investigator-initiated interventions as well as evaluations of interventions created by others (e.g., a law or a system change).

By covering both study design and statistical analysis in one book I hope to save you from having to go back and forth between a textbook on study design and one on statistics. Also, for many intervention studies, especially nonrandomized designs, understanding the statistical approach to analyzing the data is key to judging the robustness of the design. Within the statistics section I have organized the material the way that researchers think: what is the best test to perform to answer a particular question? For readers who wish to learn more about particular tests (e.g., McNemar test, mixed-effects model) I have provided references in the footnotes.

To illustrate the points in this book, I have included many examples from the medical and public health literature. Examining published articles builds on your knowledge of how to read the literature, and illustrates practical strategies to use in planning your study and analyzing the results. Also, you may find it helpful to model your study after one of the examples in the book. Given the number and range of examples I am certain you will find one that is similar to your work.

---

[1] Katz, M. H. "Interventions to increase interventions are needed." *J. Publ. Health Mgt. Pract.* **14** (2008): 224–7.

To minimize overlap between this book and my other two books: *Study Design and Statistical Analysis: A practical guide for clinicians* (Cambridge University Press, 2006) and *Multivariable Analysis: A practical guide for clinicians* (2nd edition: Cambridge University Press, 2006), I liberally cite them. Please don't see this as an expression of ego, but rather as a desire to minimize overlap. Some may prefer all the material in one text. Although that would have some advantages, it would make the books longer, more expensive, and more daunting to people new to the field. If you like this book and are interested in learning more about non-intervention studies (e.g., descriptive studies, risk-factor studies) or learning more about statistics I hope you will read these other two books.

I have benefited from reading several existing textbooks. *Experimental and Quasi-experimental Designs for Generalized Causal Inference* by W. R. Shadish, T. D. Cook and D. T. Campbell (Houghton Mifflin Company, 2002) provides a deeper theoretical review of many of the study designs included in this book. Investigators planning to conduct a clinical trial should read *Fundamentals of Clinical Trials,* by L. Friedman *et al.* (3rd edition: Springer, 1999).

I appreciate the support of my editors Richard Marley and Katie James and the staff at Cambridge University Press.

If you have any questions or suggestions for future editions, please e-mail me at mhkatz59@yahoo.com. Readers of my other two books have e-mailed me from all around the world. Writing textbooks is an arduous and lonely business. Knowing that others benefit from the books sustains me.

Introduction

1.1 Why study interventions?

Because solving problems requires interventions but not all interventions are effective!

Solving problems
requires interventions.

Let's say you are confronting the problem of obesity in your clinic or community. A necessary first step is to understand the prevalence (frequency) of obesity, the characteristics of affected individuals (e.g., age, gender, geographic location), and how severely they are affected (e.g., presence of comorbid conditions such as diabetes). A second necessary step is to identify the risk factors for obesity, especially those that are amenable to change.

But sadly too many research agendas never move beyond this second step. Investigators conclude their manuscripts with the ubiquitous and meaningless phrase: "Interventions are needed to .... ," yet the intervention is never performed. A review of bibliography sources found that only 0.4 percent of academic research focused on public health interventions.[1] Although intervention research is more common with pharmaceuticals, this research is often limited to efficacy trials conducted under conditions that cannot easily be replicated in the real world.

Develop an
intervention and
change the world!

This does not have to be the case. Developing interventions can be more fulfilling than descriptive or risk-factor studies because they can directly change the world! Interventions can be drugs or medical devices, counseling or skill-building programs for individuals or groups, laws or changes in institutional practices.

Let's return to the problem of obesity. A large body of evidence has documented a major increase in obesity rates in developed countries, with serious sequelae including type 2 diabetes. Decreased activity, larger food portions, and high caloric foods have all been shown to be risk factors for obesity.

---

[1] Millward, L., Kelly, M., and Nutbeam, D. *Public Health Intervention Research: The Evidence.* London: Health Development Agency, 2003. www.nice.org.uk/niceMedia/documents/pubhealth. interventon.pdf. Accessed 3 March, 2008.

Farley and colleagues developed a common sense intervention to increase the activity of children and thereby diminish a known risk factor for obesity: they opened a schoolyard for play during non-school hours in a low-income neighborhood in New Orleans and provided attendants to ensure children's safety.[2] The schoolyard was immediately popular: 710 children were observed in the schoolyard at least once during a 12-month period; 66% of the children were physically active when observed in the schoolyard.

To evaluate the impact of the schoolyard on the physical activity of children in the community, the investigators compared children in this community to children from a neighboring community. Prior to the opening of the schoolyard the number of children observed to be active in the intervention community was lower than in the comparison community. After the intervention, the number of children observed to be active was greater in the intervention community than in the comparison community, **not counting the children in the schoolyard.**

Besides being easy to replicate, the intervention had the advantage that it does not single out children who are obese, which may harm self-image. Rather it takes advantage of the idea that all children should be active.

To ameliorate a health problem you don't have to be the one who develops the intervention. Many useful studies have evaluated interventions that were developed by the government (e.g., laws banning smoking at workplaces) or another organization (e.g., school-based physical education). For example, Hu and colleagues assessed the impact of taxation on cigarette sales.[3] They estimated that the 25-cent tax that California added in 1989 to each pack of cigarettes resulted in a reduction of 514 million packs sold over an 18-month period. Evaluations such as this have been successful in motivating other states to add tobacco excise tax.

You may also find an unplanned opportunity, a "natural experiment," to evaluate whether a change in circumstances improves a health problem. For example, Costello and colleagues studied the impact of the opening of a casino on an Indian reservation on the mental health of Native American children.[4] The point of the casinos (the intervention) was not to improve children's mental health. However, it is known that psychopathology is higher in children from low-income families and that casinos increase the income of families living on

> Consider evaluating an intervention developed by the government or other organization.

> Keep your eyes open for a natural experiment.

[2] Farley, T. A., Meriwether, R. A., Baker, E. T., Watkins, L. T., Johnson, C. C., and Webber, L. S. "Safe play spaces to promote physical activity in inner-city children: results from a pilot study of an environmental intervention." *Am. J. Public Health* **97** (2007): 1625–31.

[3] Hu, T., Sung, H. Y., and Keeler, T. E. "Reducing cigarette consumption in California: tobacco taxes vs an anti-smoking media campaign." *Am. J. Public Health* **85** (1995): 1218–22.

[4] Costello, E. J., Compton, S. N., Keeler, G., and Angold, A. "Relationships between poverty and psychopathology: a natural experiment." *JAMA* **290** (2003): 2023–9.

a reservation. Would the presence of the casinos improve the mental health of the children?

The investigators found that after the opening of the casino the psychopathology level of the previously poor children improved to the level of the children who were never poor. The study was feasible only because a cohort study was in progress prior to the opening of the casino. The beauty of the study is that it overcomes the limitations of other possible designs: it is impossible to randomize families to higher income; a longitudinal observational cohort study looking at the connection between income and children's mental health would have the challenge of separating the impact of income gains from the impact of the factors that led to the gain in income (e.g., new job, second parent working).

1.2　How can you tell whether an intervention is effective?

It is not always easy! Of course, if you develop a new treatment for rabies (a disease that is almost uniformly fatal without prompt treatment) and your first ten patients all survive, you may have enough evidence to prove your case. But, most of the health problems that plague the twenty-first century world do not have a single cause; most of the outcomes don't occur quickly or predictably; and no intervention is expected to be near 100% effective. Rather, problems like obesity, violence or substance abuse have multiple interrelated causes; outcomes occur over a period of years; and an intervention that reduced the prevalence of any of these conditions by 15% would be heralded as a major breakthrough.

There are a wide variety of study designs available for evaluating the effectiveness of interventions, each with their own advantages and disadvantages.[5] Studies may be randomized or nonrandomized, prospective or retrospective, clustered or nonclustered. Investigators may use complicated analytic tools such as time-series analysis or multivariable modeling, or simply compare percentages. Regardless of what study designs and analytic tools are employed, determining whether the intervention works will be based on answering one (or more) of the following three questions:

1　Is the post-intervention assessment significantly different from the pre-intervention assessment?

---

[5] The term evaluation encompasses a broad set of activities including assessing whether a problem exists, how well a program is functioning (e.g., number of clients being served, length of time it takes to serve a client, client satisfaction with the service), what the program costs, etc. The focus of this book is the efficacy or effectiveness of the intervention. For an excellent book on the full spectrum of evaluation activities see: Berk, R. A. and Rossi, P. H. *Thinking about Program Evaluation 2.* Thousand Oaks: Sage Publications, 1999; also Shadish, W. R. "The common threads in program evaluation." *Prev Chronic Dis* **391** (2006): A03 at http://www.pubmedcentral.nih.gov/articlerender.fcgi?tool=pubmed&pubmedid=16356356.

2 Is the change between the pre-intervention and the post-intervention assessment of the intervention group significantly different than that of the comparison group?

3 Is the outcome for the intervention group significantly different than for the comparison group?

In the next section I will review the data elements you will need to answer each of these questions. Following that I will discuss development of interventions (Chapter 2), evaluation of interventions (Chapter 3), and then compare randomized designs (Chapter 4) to nonrandomized designs (Chapter 5). In Chapter 6 I will return to how to answer these three questions from a statistical point of view.

1.2.A Is the post-intervention assessment significantly different from the pre-intervention assessment?

An intuitively simple way of determining whether an intervention works is to assess a group of people prior to it (pre-intervention) and again after it (post-intervention) (Figure 1.1). This is referred to as a one-group pre-intervention versus post-intervention design.

> Longitudinal cohort studies repeatedly assess the same individuals over time.

If you are assessing the same individuals on more than one occasion, your study is a longitudinal cohort study. If you are sampling from the same population but not necessarily the same individuals on more than one occasion, you are performing a serial cross-sectional study. By definition one-group pre-intervention versus post-intervention designs are nonrandomized designs because you need at least two groups to randomize assignment.

> Serial cross-sectional studies repeatedly sample from the same population over time.

Regardless of whether you are assessing the same individuals over time, or samples of the same population over time, you will be testing the null hypothesis; in this case, that there is no difference between the two assessments. If the difference between the pre-intervention and post-intervention assessments is sufficiently great that it is unlikely that the difference could have occurred by chance alone, you will consider the alternative hypothesis: that the intervention worked. If the pre-intervention and post-intervention assessments are similar, you will conclude that the null hypothesis was correct: the intervention did not work.

Let's look at a very important intervention evaluated with a one-group pre-intervention versus post-intervention design. Pronovost and colleagues designed an intervention to decrease catheter-related blood infections among patients cared for in the intensive care unit.[6] The intervention included

---

[6] Pronovost, P., Needham, D., Berenholtz, S., *et al.* "An intervention to decrease catheter-related bloodstream infections in the ICU." *N. Engl. J. Med.* **355** (2006): 2725–32.

Introduction

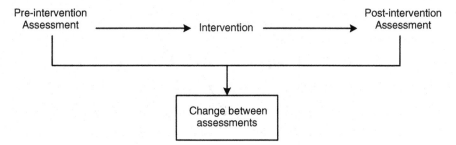

Figure 1.1   Schematic of one-group pre-intervention versus post-intervention design.

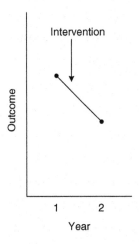

Figure 1.2   Hypothetical data with a pre-intervention and a post-intervention assessment.

strategies to increase hand-washing by medical personnel, use of barrier precautions, antibacterial cleaning of the catheter site, avoiding use of the femoral site, and removing unnecessary catheters.

Three months after the intervention there were significantly fewer infections (0 infections per 1000 catheter days) than before the intervention (2.7 infections per 1000 catheter days). The probability was small ($P \leq 0.002$) that the change in the infection rate between the pre-intervention and the post-intervention assessments occurred by chance.

To appreciate one of the weaknesses of a pre-intervention versus post-intervention evaluation such as this one, look at the hypothetical data in Figure 1.2. It appears that there has been a major drop in outcomes (e.g., infection, cancer, heart disease) following institution of an intervention.

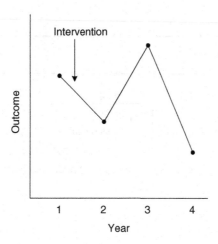

Figure 1.3   Hypothetical data with a pre-intervention assessment and three post-intervention assessments.

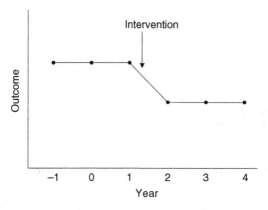

Figure 1.4   Hypothetical data with three pre-intervention assessments and three post-intervention assessments.

Before concluding that the intervention worked, look at Figure 1.3. It is the continuation of the same study. You can see that outcomes were back up by year 3 and back down by year 4. Remember: two points do not make a trend.

One way to improve the strength of a single group pre-intervention versus post-intervention design is to get additional data points. For example, if the frequency of outcome had been measured several times prior to the intervention and was stable, and then changed precipitously following the intervention, and the change was sustained at several points after the intervention, as shown in Figure 1.4, you would have much greater confidence that the decrease in outcome was due to the intervention.

> Two points do not make a trend.

Table 1.1. Rate of catheter-related infection at baseline, during the intervention, and after the intervention.

	Rate of infection (95% confidence intervals)	P value for comparison with baseline rate
Baseline	2.7 (0.6–4.8)	–
During intervention	1.6 (0–4.4)	≤0.05
After intervention		
0–3 mo	0 (0–3.0)	≤0.002
4–6 mo	0 (0–2.7)	≤0.002
7–9 mo	0 (0–2.1)	≤0.002
10–12 mo	0 (0–1.9)	≤0.002
13–15 mo	0 (0–1.6)	≤0.002
16–18 mo	0 (0–2.4)	≤0.002

Data from Pronovost, P., *et al.* "An intervention to decrease catheter-related bloodstream infections in the ICU." *N. Engl. J. Med.* **355** (2006): 2725–32.

In the case of the study to decrease infections in the ICU, the investigators had only one measurement of infection prior to the intervention, but they had additional data points: one during the implementation period and five additional points in the post-intervention period (Table 1.1). These data points increase confidence that the intervention worked. When you have lots of consecutive data points over a period of time you can analyze your data using time series analysis (Chapter 8).

However, no matter how many data points you have prior to, during, and after an intervention, with only one group your study has a serious limitation: there is always the possibility that any observed change occurred for a reason other than the intervention. Returning to the example of the study of catheter-related infections in the ICU, perhaps infections decreased due to media attention on hospital infection rates or changes in physician prescribing practices with respect to antibiotics. To overcome this limitation we need a design that includes a comparison group. This design is discussed in the next subsection.

1.2.B Is the change between the pre-intervention and the post-intervention assessment of the intervention group significantly greater (lesser) than that of the comparison group?

Adding one or more comparison groups to a pre-intervention versus post-intervention assessment results in a stronger evaluation design than having a single group. If the subjects are assigned by random to the groups and the subjects are followed prospectively, you have a randomized controlled trial

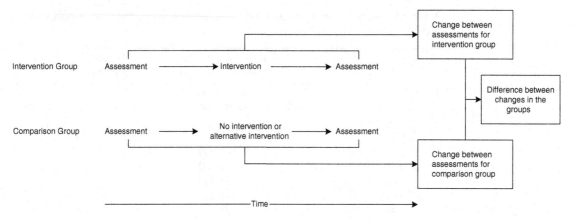

Figure 1.5   Schematic diagram of a pre-intervention versus post-intervention design with
comparison group.

(Chapter 4). There are also a number of ways of assembling a comparable control group without randomization (Chapter 5).

Whether the comparison group is assigned randomly or not, the major question is whether the change that occurs between the pre-intervention and the post-intervention assessment is greater (lesser) than the change over the same period of time in a comparison population (Figure 1.5).

To illustrate the benefits of adding a comparison group to a pre-intervention versus post-intervention assessment, let's look at a study evaluating whether providing hospitals with confidential information on their performance improves the care of patients having coronary artery bypass grafting (CABG).[7] The intervention was performed at 20 hospitals in Alabama.

In Table 1.2 you can see the impact of the intervention on four important process measures. Following the intervention the rate of internal mammary artery use, the percentage of patients discharged on aspirin, and the percentage of patients who were intubated for less than 6 hours increased, and the median time patients were intubated decreased. But as with the study of ICU catheter infections, is it possible that these changes occurred for some reason other than the intervention? Indeed, three and a half years passed between the start of the pre-intervention assessment and the end of the post-intervention assessment. Perhaps improvements in surgical technique or medical practice during these years are the actual cause of the observed improvement in practice.

The investigators addressed this concern by including CABG patients from a comparison state. As you can see in Table 1.3 the changes over time were more

[7] Holman, W. L., Allman, R. M., Sansom, M., *et al.* "Alabama coronary artery bypass grafting project: results of a statewide quality improvement initiative." *JAMA* **285** (2001): 3003–10.

Table 1.2. Impact of a quality improvement program in Alabama hospitals.

Measure	Pre-intervention	Post-intervention	P value
Internal mammary artery use, %	73	84	≤0.001
Aspirin therapy, %	88	92	≤0.001
Intubation time, median, h	12	7	≤0.001
Intubation <6 h, %	9	41	≤0.001

Data from: Holman, W. L., *et al.* "Alabama coronary artery bypass grafting project: results of a statewide quality improvement initiative." *JAMA* **285** (2001): 3003–10.

Table 1.3. Quality indicators for CABG surgery in Alabama compared to another state.

Measure	Alabama		Comparison state		P value for difference between states
	Pre-intervention	Post-intervention	Baseline	Follow-up	
Internal mammary artery use, %	73	84	48	55	= 0.001
Aspirin therapy, %	88	92	86	82	<0.001
Intubation time, median, h	12	7	7	8	<0.001
Intubation <6 h, %	9	41	40	39	<0.001

Data from: Holman, W. L., *et al.* "Alabama coronary artery bypass grafting project: results of a statewide quality improvement initiative." *JAMA* **285** (2001): 3003–10.

favorable in the intervention state (Alabama) than in the comparison state. Temporal improvements in medical practice would have likely influenced the outcomes in the comparison state as well.

Note also from Table 1.3 the importance of having two measurements from both of the states. If you had only the second measurements for the median intubation time and for the percentage of patients who were intubated for less than six hours, you might conclude that there was no difference between the two states. If you had only the second measurements for internal mammary artery use you would think that the intervention was a much greater success that it was – even before the intervention, the use of the internal mammary artery as part of the CABG procedure was substantially higher in Alabama hospitals than in the comparison state.

Although the inclusion of a comparison group (in this case concurrent controls) greatly strengthens the model, there remains an important potential weakness. Is the comparison group comparable to the intervention group? As you can see from Table 1.4, patients from the intervention group and the comparison group are similar on most characteristics at both baseline and follow-up assessments. Nonetheless there are differences (for example, the percentage with left main disease is lower in Alabama than in the comparison state).

Table 1.4. Characteristics of patients receiving a CABG in Alabama compared to patients receiving a CABG in another state

Characteristics	Alabama		Comparison state	
	Pre-intervention	Post-intervention	Baseline	Follow-up
Patients	4090	1694	2288	926
Mean age, y	69.9	70.7	70.6	71.4
Male, %	65	55	66	66
White, %	91	91	94	93
CAD				
Left main, %	16	19	23	27
MI within 3 days, %	9	14	8	9
MI within 6 months, %	22	26	21	24
CHF	16	22	12	19
Poor LVF, %	26	29	20	19
Cardiogenic shock, %	3	3	3	2
COPD, %	25	30	23	31
Diabetes mellitus, %	29	32	27	32
Dialysis, %	2	1	1	2

Data from: Holman, W. L., *et al.* "Alabama coronary artery bypass grafting project: results of a statewide quality improvement initiative." *JAMA* **285** (2001): 3003–10.

Could some other difference between Alabama hospitals and those in the comparison state explain the differences that we are attributing to Alabama's intervention? Yes. The only way to be certain that there are no important differences between the intervention and the comparison group is to randomize assignment to the groups (Chapter 4).

Still, it is important to note that this intervention, which had an important impact, would have been very difficult to perform using a randomized design. Randomization of individual patients would have been impossible because the intervention was being performed on the level of physicians and hospitals.

A clustered randomization design (Section 4.5), where the hospitals were randomized to be in the intervention, would have been superior from a design point of view. However, this study was possible because of a statewide initiative in Alabama to improve the care of patients receiving CABG in all hospitals and had the cooperation of the state peer review organization. The comparison state only had to agree to release medical record information.

Randomizing hospitals may have created another problem: it may have increased the diffusion of the intervention to non-intervention hospitals because physicians often work at more than one hospital and share information through local and state professional associations. Diffusion of the intervention would have been good for care of patients receiving CABG but would have made it difficult to demonstrate that the intervention worked. Having the intervention performed in one state and compared to performance in another state minimized contamination of the comparison community with the intervention (Section 3.6).

A final note on this study: you may have been surprised when you saw from the *N* of patients listed in Table 1.4 that the same patients are not in both the baseline and follow-up. That's because this is a serial cross-sectional study. The advantages and disadvantages of serial cross-sectional designs are discussed in Section 3.7 and the statistics for analyzing serial cross-sectional data are reviewed in Section 6.3 and 6.5.

1.2.C Is the outcome for the intervention group significantly different than for the comparison group?

Sometimes we need to evaluate an intervention for which no pre-intervention measurement has been made. For example, laws and organizational practices are often changed without anyone planning an evaluation. With ingenuity it may be possible to identify some pre-intervention measures, perhaps by identifying a prospective cohort that was operating before the intervention, or assembling a retrospective cohort by using existing records, such as an electronic health record (see Section 3.4 for suggestions). But what if you cannot identify any pre-intervention measurements? In such circumstances it may be possible to compare a post-intervention assessment to an assessment of a comparison group (Figure 1.6).

For example, beginning in 1979, a number of local laws were passed restricting tobacco smoking in public workplaces (e.g., restaurants, stores) in California. Moskowitz and colleagues evaluated whether these ordinances resulted in

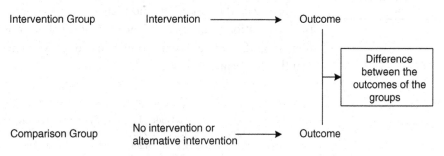

Figure 1.6   Schematic of a design comparing the outcome between the intervention and comparison groups.

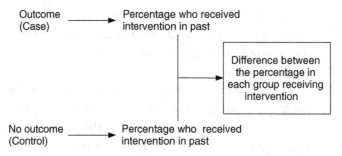

Figure 1.7   Schematic diagram of a case-control study to determine whether the outcome is associated with receipt of the intervention.

people quitting smoking.[8] In 1990 they performed a cross-sectional survey of adult indoor workers. Among persons working in areas with strong no-smoking ordinances 26% of smokers quit in the prior six months, while only 19% of smokers quit in areas with no ordinances. The probability that this difference occurred by chance was small ($P < 0.001$).

A major weakness of this design is that without a pre-intervention assessment, we cannot test for or adjust for pre-existing differences between the groups. Perhaps persons living in the areas where tobacco smoking was restricted were more likely to quit smoking anyway, for some reason other than the workplace ordinances. For example, maybe there is stronger community pressure to not smoke and that is the reason the bans were passed and people quit. This is a fair criticism, and one not easily refuted. This is why intervention studies without a pre-intervention measurement are much weaker. Nonetheless, the study added to a growing body of research indicating that smoking bans have positive impacts on community health.[9]

Another way to evaluate an intervention without a pre-intervention assessment is to perform a case-control study.[10] With a case-control study, you identify people with a disease or condition and a control group of persons without the disease or the condition, and then assess what percent of each group had the intervention (Figure 1.7). If the percentage of persons having the intervention is significantly different in the two groups, you have suggestive evidence that the intervention works.

| Case-control studies can be used to evaluate an intervention without a pre-intervention assessment. |

---

[8] Moskowitz, J. M., Lin, Z., and Hudes, E. S. "The impact of workplace smoking ordinances in California on smoking cessation." *Am. J. Public Health* **90** (2000): 757–61.

[9] Pell, J. P., Haw, S., Cobbe, S., *et al.* "Smoke-free legislation and hospitalizations for acute coronary syndrome." *N. Engl. J. Med.* **359** (2008): 482–91.

[10] Case-control methods may be more familiar to you from studies of risk factors/exposures of disease, but the method works for evaluating interventions as well.

Table 1.5. Effect of environmental control measures on the risk of homicide in North Carolina workplaces.

Control Measures	Cases (N = 105)	Controls (N = 210)	Odds Ratio (95% confidence interval)	
			Unadjusted	Adjusted*
Lighting and visibility				
Bright lighting outside building	28%	33%	0.8 (0.5–1.3)	0.5 (0.3–1.0)
Bright lighting inside during work hours	57%	64%	0.7 (0.5–1.2)	0.7 (0.3–1.3)
Bright lighting inside before/ after hours	37%	41%	0.8 (0.5–1.4)	0.9 (0.4–1.7)
Workers visible from outside	61%	60%	1.1 (0.7–1.7)	1.0 (0.5–1.9)
Access				
Barrier between workers and public	83%	88%	0.6 (0.3–1.3)	0.6 (0.2–1.8)
Security and surveillance devices				
Video cameras	25%	16%	1.8 (1.0–3.2)	1.3 (0.6–2.8)
Alarms	19%	26%	0.7 (0.4–1.2)	0.5 (0.2–1.0)
Mirrors	30%	21%	1.6 (0.9–2.8)	0.8 (0.4–1.8)
Other devices	24%	25%	1.0 (0.6–1.7)	0.8 (0.4–1.7)
Cash storage				
Drop box	21%	21%	1.0 (0.5–2.0)	0.5 (0.2–1.3)
Safe with worker access	46%	48%	0.9 (0.5–1.6)	1.3 (0.6–2.9)
> Five environmental control measures	34%	40%	0.8 (0.5–1.3)	0.5 (0.2–1.0)

* Adjusted for a priori high-risk industry, residential or industrial location, open Saturdays, workforce race and sex, relocated or opened in last 2 years. Ns vary for the different measures; see original article for actual Ns.
Data from: Loomis, D., *et al.* "Effectiveness of safety measures recommended for prevention of workplace homicide." *JAMA* **287** (2002): 1011–7.

For example, Loomis and colleagues used a case-control study to evaluate the effectiveness of safety measures for preventing homicides at workplaces.[11] Using a statewide database from the medical examiner system they identified 105 homicides that occurred at a work site. Next they identified 210 workplaces from a business phone listing where no homicide had occurred.[12] To determine whether the safety measures were effective in preventing homicides, they asked informants at the workplaces whether a variety of security measures were in place during the month the homicide had occurred (for cases) and for the same

[11] Loomis, D., Marshall, S. W., Wolf, S. H., Runyan, C. W., and Butts, J. D. "Effectiveness of safety measures recommended for prevention of workplace homicide." *JAMA* **287** (2002): 1011–7.

[12] The cases and controls in this study are workplaces rather than people because the purpose of the study was to see whether there were different security measures at workplaces where there were no homicides.

month for the controls. Cases and controls were then compared on whether the safety measure was in place. As you can see in Table 1.5, having bright light outside the building, having alarms, and having greater than five environmental control measures were associated with a lower likelihood of a homicide (last column) after adjustment for a variety of factors.

A major limitation of case-control studies such as this is that you are relying on reporting of the past by cases and controls, and people's memories can be affected by events that have occurred to them. For example, informants at workplaces that experienced a homicide might feel that their workplace was unsafe (since a homicide had occurred) and under-report workplace safety measures. This problem is eliminated in nested case-control studies (case-control studies that are performed within an ongoing cohort) because cases and controls are interviewed prior to the development of the disease or condition. But in the real world there are circumstances where no pre-intervention measurement exists and you have to do your best to evaluate the intervention.

2

Interventions

2.1 What type of interventions are commonly evaluated in medicine and public health?

A wide variety of interventions can be evaluated. Table 2.1 is meant to be illustrative, perhaps even inspirational, but not exhaustive.

I will discuss more about how to design interventions in the next section and then in Chapter 3 take up the question of how to evaluate interventions.

2.2 How do I design an intervention?

The first step in designing an intervention is to have a thorough understanding of the problem you are trying to solve. Read the published literature. Identifying published articles has been made easy and free by PubMed (http://www.ncbi.nlm.nih.gov/Pubmed). Perform a Google search as well because sometimes interesting work is unpublished but available on the net. Talk to others in your field and on the ground. Involving community experts and stakeholders is a great way of learning more about a problem and potential solutions (Section 3.1).

> **TIP**
>
> Use PubMed to identify the published research and a Google search to find unpublished work.

The process of researching the problem will likely also lead you to solutions that have already been tried. When possible, build on what has already been learned. Although the universe of possible interventions is broad, I offer the following considerations that I believe will increase the chance that your intervention will be a success (Table 2.2).

2.2.A Base intervention on theory and/or pathophysiology

An intervention is more likely to be effective if it is grounded in theory. For example, Hawkins and colleagues developed an intervention to decrease adolescent high-risk behaviors such as violence, crime, substance abuse, and sexual activity.[1] The intervention was based on the social development

---

[1] Hawkins, J. D., Catalano, R. F., Kosterman, R., Abbott, R., and Hill, K. G. "Preventing adolescent health-risk behaviors by strengthening protection during childhood." *Arch. Pediatr. Adolesc. Med.* **153** (1999): 226–34.

Table 2.1. Types of interventions that can be evaluated.

Type of intervention	Example	Advantages	Disadvantages
Investigator-developed interventions	Develop an intervention to increase exercise among young people and evaluate whether youth exposed to the intervention exercise more than those who are not exposed.	Can ensure that design of intervention and evaluation fit well together.	Most expensive, need to consent people for the intervention as well as for the evaluation.
Quality improvement program	Evaluate infection rates after placing antimicrobial gel dispensers outside patient rooms.	No need to create or pay for intervention; may not need to consent participants (depending on the outcome measure used).	Not possible to randomize participants; may be difficult to identify a comparable group that has not experienced the intervention.
Introduction of a new medication, procedure, or device into practice	Evaluate whether drug-eluting stents are superior to regular stents.	No need to create or pay for intervention.	The first group to receive an intervention may differ from others (e.g., may be sicker); also subject to survival bias (i.e., subjects have to live long enough to get treatment).
Change in style or practice	Evaluate whether adding menu labeling improves diets.	No need to create or pay for intervention.	May only have historic controls available.
Evaluating a law or government regulation	Evaluate smoking rates following passage of smoking bans.	No need to create or pay for intervention; laws and regulations often have very broad implications and can be implemented in other localities.	Generally have to rely on administrative data for pre-law/regulation data.
Natural or man-made occurrence	Gambling casinos open on an Indian reservation.	Natural experiments can produce conditions that would be unethical to create as part of a research project.	Cannot plan for natural experiments.

model. According to the model, specific social factors (e.g., parental involvement, social participation skills) influence children's bonds to their school; strong bonds to school, in turn, protect youth against engaging in problematic behaviors.

> An intervention is more likely to be effective if it is grounded in theory.

Based on this theory, the intervention targeted teachers, parents, and the children themselves during early childhood years (grades one to six). Teachers

Table 2.2. Considerations for developing interventions.

Consideration	Importance
Base intervention on theory and/or pathophysiology	Increases chances of intervention succeeding, increases chance that positive findings are real, improves generalizability.
Build on prior experience	Allows for sample size calculation, identifies potential weaknesses that can be addressed prior to initiation of study, increases chances of intervention succeeding, increases chance that positive findings are real.
Make your intervention practical Cost Availability of expertise Willingness of persons to participate	Determines likelihood that intervention will be sustained or translated into standard practice.

were instructed on methods of increasing the involvement of children in the class and on helping children learn better ways of interacting with each other. Children received social instruction in grade six. Parents were offered classes in child behavior appropriate to the age of their children.

The investigators found that children who had received the intervention were less likely to report violent behavior and heavy drinking by the age of 18 years than children who had not participated in the intervention.

Grounding an intervention in a theory increases our confidence that the result is not spurious. Why? Because our expectation prior to the study (in Bayesian terms, the prior probability of success) is higher that the intervention will work if it is based on an accurate theory. Conversely, if an intervention is not based on a theory or prior experience, we worry more that a statistically significant finding might be spurious.

Grounding an intervention in a theory also increases the generalizability of a study result. Generalizability refers to the likelihood that the intervention would have a similar affect among other persons in other settings. How does theory improve generalizability? If a theory is true then changes in populations and settings should not change the overall impact of the intervention. (Think of the theory of relativity – it applies throughout the universe.)

As has been pointed out by others,[2] the major limitation to basing interventions on theory is how few theories there are that can explain complex human behavior.

> Grounding an intervention in a theory increases our confidence that the result is not spurious.

> Generalizability refers to the likelihood that the intervention would have a similar affect among other persons in other settings.

[2] Berk, R. A. and Rossi, P. H. *Thinking about Program Evaluation 2*. Sage: Thousand Oaks, 1999.

With medical studies the "theory" is the pathophysiology of a disease.

For most medical studies, the "theory" is the pathophysiology of a disease. To the extent that the impact of the intervention on the physiology of the disease can be predicted ahead of the study, the intervention is more likely to be successful and the findings of your study (assuming they are in the predicted direction) are more likely to be believed.

For example the ADVANCE trial was designed to test whether a combination of an ACE-inhibitor and a thiazide diuretic could reduce vascular complications among type 2 diabetics.[3] Although most studies aiming at preventing the vascular complications of diabetes focus on reducing glucose levels, the investigators knew that reducing blood pressure also reduces vascular complications. The average systolic blood pressure drop was 5.6 mmHg among patients randomized to receive an ACE-inhibitor. Of greater significance, the investigators found that major macrovascular and microvascular complications were reduced by 9% among those randomized to receive an ACE-inhibitor and a thiazide diuretic compared to those randomized to placebo. The effect of ACE-inhibitors on vascular complications among diabetics in the ADVANCE trial was so strong that it has become standard practice to treat all diabetics with evidence of renal disease with an ACE-inhibitor even if they are not hypertensive.

Of course, just because you think that you understand how an intervention would improve a disease is no guarantee that you are right. For example, there were detailed physiologic explanations of why estrogen would be expected to decrease the incidence of heart disease in women, including that estrogen is known to decrease low-density lipoproteins (the bad kind of cholesterol), increase high-density lipoproteins (the good kind of cholesterol), improve endothelial vascular function, and lower fibrinogen and plasminogen levels.[4] These explanations were in turn supported by a number of observational studies showing that estrogen decreased heart disease in women.[5] Unfortunately, when a large blinded multicenter randomized placebo-controlled trial was conducted, estrogen plus progestin increased cardiovascular disease.[6]

[3] Bakris, G. L. and Berkwits, M. "Trials that matter: The effect of a fixed-dose combination of an angiotensin-converting enzyme inhibitor and a diuretic on the complications of type 2 diabetes." *Ann. Intern. Med.* **148** (2008): 400–1. Patel, A., ADVANCE Collaborative Group. "Effects of a fixed combination of perindopril and indapamide on macrovascular and microvascular outcomes in patients with type 2 diabetes mellitus (the ADVANCE trial): A randomized controlled trial." *Lancet* **370** (2007): 829–40.

[4] Manson, J. E. and Martin, K. A. "Postmenopausal hormone-replacement therapy." *N. Engl. J. Med.* **345** (2001): 34–40.

[5] Grodstein, F., Clarkson, T. B., and Manson, J. E. "Understanding the divergent data on postmenopausal hormone therapy." *N. Engl. J. Med.* **348** (2003): 645–50.

[6] Writing Group for the Women's Health Initiative Investigators. "Risks and benefits of estrogen plus progestin in healthy postmenopausal women: principal results from the Women's Health Initiative randomized controlled trial." *JAMA* **288** (2002): 321–33.

2.2.B Build on prior experience

An intervention that has succeeded previously is more likely to be successful. Of course, we wouldn't have major breakthroughs if we only extended previously successful interventions.

> For novel interventions conduct a pilot study before performing a full-scale implementation.

If your intervention is novel, conduct a pilot study before performing a full-scale implementation. There are several reasons for this. First, as a practical matter, it is impossible to conduct a sample size calculation (Section 3.12) unless you can estimate the effectiveness of an intervention. Second, pilot studies are particularly helpful in pretesting measurement instruments and recruitment strategies. Third, a pilot study is likely to help you recognize potential weaknesses in your design. For example, you may find that you have an unacceptably high drop-out rate in the intervention arm. This may lead you to modify the intervention. Or perhaps you will find that your outcome measurement does not fully capture the effects of the intervention.

2.2.C Make your intervention practical

Ultimately the best reason for developing and evaluating an intervention is to identify those that should be broadly implemented.

The traditional paradigm for developing, evaluating, implementing, and translating interventions is shown in Figure 2.1. In the first stage an intervention is tested to see whether it works in a research setting (efficacy trial). The teaching has been that in an efficacy trial the intervention should be delivered in a uniform fashion by trained research personnel. Subjects are enrolled, closely followed, and may receive stipends for their participation.

> Efficacy trials test interventions in research settings.

Efficacy trials typically enroll homogeneous populations because subjects who are atypical (e.g., over 90 years of age) may respond differently to the treatment. Related to this, many efficacy trials exclude persons who are very ill or thought to be at greater risk of harm from the intervention or who have a deficit (e.g., dementia) that results in their being unable to comply with all aspects of

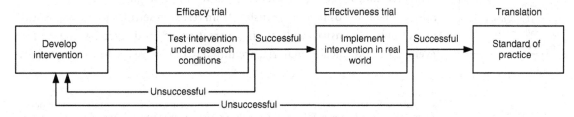

Figure 2.1   Traditional paradigm for developing, evaluating, and translating an intervention.

the study. Because the focus of an efficacy trial is to eliminate confounding, it is expected that the controls will be randomized.

Following the traditional paradigm, if an intervention works in an efficacy trial, it should then be tested in "real-world" conditions (effectiveness trial). In an effectiveness trial subjects may be enrolled or passively followed. Effectiveness trials should include a broad range of subjects and the practitioners who deliver the intervention should be similar in skills to the people who will be implementing the intervention in the real world.

Effectiveness trials may randomize subjects to an intervention and a control group, or may have a nonrandomized comparison group, or may have no comparison group at all. The reason you may not need a control group is that once you have proven that an intervention is more efficacious than standard treatment in a randomized trial, you can focus your efforts in the effectiveness trial on simply demonstrating that your intervention works as well in real-world conditions as it did in the trial.

If an intervention is found to work in an effectiveness trial, then it can be translated into the standard of practice.

There are several problems with this paradigm. First, those interventions that are most likely to succeed in efficacy trials are not necessarily the same interventions that are likely to succeed in real-world conditions. For example, interventions that are expensive, time-consuming, or require highly trained staff may be very successful in an efficacy study but unsuccessful in an effectiveness study. Glasgow and colleagues have pointed out that this has resulted in a disconnect in what was supposed to be a linear transition between efficacy and effectiveness studies.[7] The authors suggest a number of ways to close the gap. Without detailing their thoughtful argument, which I hope you will read, much of what they are calling for is performing intervention studies at both the efficacy and effectiveness stages that are likely to be implementable.

To be certain that you do not develop and evaluate an intervention that will never be adopted consider: expense, expertise, and interest in participation among those needing the intervention. Further suggestions on how to translate your research findings into standard practice are included in Chapter 10.

Interventions that are extremely expensive or that require expertise not generally available are difficult to translate from research settings to the real world. For example, expensive medications to treat common diseases in the underdeveloped world, such as malaria, are unlikely to receive broad use, especially

---

| Effectiveness trials test interventions in real-world settings. |

| Interventions most likely to succeed in efficacy trials are not necessarily most likely to succeed in real-world conditions. |

| Expensive and/or resource-intensive interventions are hard to implement, especially in resource-poor areas. |

---

[7] Glasgow, R. E., Lichtenstein, E., and Marcus, A. C. "Why don't we see more translation of health promotion research to practice? Rethinking the efficacy-to-effectiveness transition." *Am. J. Public Health* **93** (2003): 1261–7.

if they require technologically sophisticated laboratory studies to monitor for toxicity.

Some interventions are difficult to translate because a large number of persons who need the intervention are ineligible to participate. People may be ineligible to participate because it requires them to be in a particular state of health (e.g., not be housebound) or have certain life circumstances (e.g., telephones). For example, chronic disease management interventions involving mail or phone reminders would not be practical for caring for the homeless.

> If a large proportion of eligible subjects are excluded from an intervention trial it is probably difficult to implement it in a real-world setting.

One helpful indication of the practicality of an intervention is the proportion of potential subjects who are excluded from the study. Interventions that exclude a large percentage of persons who need the intervention are not very practical, even when they are effective. For example, Wolchik and colleagues developed two theory-grounded interventions to decrease mental health and behavioral problems among adolescents with divorced parents.[8] One intervention entailed mothers participating in 11 group sessions and two individual sessions; the other intervention involved these same 13 sessions for the mothers and another 11 group sessions for the children; the control group received books on postdivorce adjustment.

The investigators found that compared to adolescents in the control group, those in the two intervention groups had fewer symptoms of mental disorders, and less alcohol and drug use six years after the intervention. These are important benefits and it is heartening that the effect was long-lasting. But will the intervention be widely implemented? I think not.

Here's the reason. Of 1816 families randomly selected from divorce-court records or identified via referral or response to the media, 1331 were contacted by phone. Of these only 671 met the inclusion criteria of the study (e.g., neither the mother nor any child in the family needed treatment for a mental health problem; mother had no live-in boyfriend or plans to remarry during the study; mother and child were fluent in English). Of these 671 families, 453 completed the recruitment visit, 341 agreed to participate, and 315 completed the pretest. At the pretest 49 more were found to be ineligible and 26 refused to participate after the pretest, resulting in 240 families being randomized to one of the three groups; an additional 26 families withdrew after being assigned. Therefore, only 214 (12%) of divorced families with children who were originally identified actually completed the trial.

For this trial, families were paid for their participation (although not for the actual counseling sessions); in the real world people are not offered financial

---

[8] Wolchik, S. A., Sandler, I. N., Millsap, R. E., *et al.* "Six-year follow-up of preventive interventions for children of divorce." *JAMA* **288** (2002): 1874–81.

incentives, which may result in lower participation. So while the evaluation demonstrates compelling benefits for those who participate, it is an open question how many divorced families would participate if it were available. Even if we had a strategy to convince all divorced families to participate, the results of the study cannot be generalized to all divorced families because only a small percentage of identified families participated.

Although the cost of the program is not listed, it is likely to be very expensive because it included a large number of sessions and extensively trained master's degree-level clinicians led the sessions. Even if enough funding were provided, it may not be possible to identify a sufficient number of master's degree clinicians to deliver the intervention.

My comments about this study may seem critical, but I specifically chose it to illustrate the challenges of translating research findings because I thought it was a good intervention for a common problem with a strong outcome. Although it can be difficult to know how easily an intervention will translate into everyday practice, consider issues of translation right from the start and try to create an intervention that can be broadly implemented.

Evaluating an intervention

3.1 How do I engage stakeholders?

If you have developed an intervention, you have ideally involved stakeholders in the creation of it. But whether you are evaluating an intervention you developed or whether you are evaluating an intervention developed by someone else, it is critical to engage stakeholders.

| Engage stakeholders. |

Depending on the program you are evaluating, the stakeholders may be community members, businesses, advocacy groups, patients, teachers, parents, or elected officials. Stakeholders are an invaluable part of any evaluation. They can lead you to the important questions, problems, and pitfalls that will otherwise ambush the unsuspecting researcher; they can help you to develop your intervention, pretest it, enroll subjects, and obtain cooperation from necessary institutions, including writing support letters for funders; and they can help you to interpret your data and disseminate your results.

| Form a community advisory committee. |

It is often helpful to establish a community advisory committee for your project, as well as having open forums so that persons who are interested but don't have the time to participate on a regular basis can be involved. Monthly meetings with food are a good way to keep ideas and information flowing back and forth.[1] If you receive funding for your study, provide stipends for committee members; it demonstrates that you value their time equally to your own.

3.2 What data should I collect for evaluating my intervention?

If you are designing an intervention you have a tremendous advantage over those who attempt to evaluate interventions they have not created (Section 3.4). You have the opportunity to embed the evaluation within the intervention.

| Collect data prior to the intervention, during the intervention, and after the intervention. |

At a minimum, collect data prior to the intervention, during the intervention, and after the intervention (Table 3.1). Often it is better to collect multiple

---

[1] For more on engaging stakeholders and other helpful pointers on conducting evaluations see: CDC. "Framework for program evaluation in public health." *MMWR* **48** (1999) (RR11): 1–40. www.cdc. gov/mmwr/preview/mmwrhtml/rr4811a1.htm.

Table 3.1. Important data collection points for evaluating interventions.

Needed data points	Reason
Multiple measurements of the outcome prior to the intervention.	Determine whether there is a trend prior to the intervention being implemented.
Multiple measurements of the outcome during the intervention.	Determine a dose response to the intervention.
Multiple measurements of the outcome after the intervention.	Determine whether the impact of the intervention wanes, stays the same, or grows.

data points at these three critical points. Multiple data points prior to the intervention determine whether there is a temporal trend prior to the intervention (e.g., perhaps hospital infections were already decreasing prior to your intervention); multiple data points during the intervention provide a measure of dose response (e.g., as participants have greater exposure to the intervention is there greater change?). Multiple data points after the intervention tell you whether the impact of the intervention diminishes, increases, or stays the same over time.

3.3 How do I choose a control group for evaluating my intervention?

Besides planning your data collection points, another major planning issue is to determine whether you will have a control group. Although important evaluations can be conducted without a control group using a one-group pre-intervention versus post-intervention design (Section 1.2.A), having a control group strengthens all designs.

The different types of control group with their advantages and disadvantages are listed in Table 3.2.

> Only randomization can produce controls that are unbiased.

The best control group is created by randomizing all eligible subjects and observing the controls concurrently. This ensures that group membership is unbiased. However, at times it may not be ethical or feasible to withhold the intervention from some of the subjects (e.g., parents may not consent to their children being randomized to receive or not receive an intervention designed to prevent substance use). Even if it is ethical, it may be hard to motivate people to remain in a trial where they know they are not receiving an intervention (this latter problem can be minimized in medication studies where a placebo can be provided – placebos are harder to construct for other types of interventions).

> Waiting-list controls are a good way of guaranteeing that all subjects can receive the intervention while still performing randomization.

Waiting-list controls are a practical compromise when it is not possible to randomize subjects to receive or not receive an intervention. Subjects may be randomized to receive an intervention or to be a waiting-list control with the promise that the controls will receive the intervention as soon as the first group

Table 3.2. Advantages and disadvantages of different types of controls.

Type of control	Advantages	Disadvantages
Randomized control	Groups are comparable on measured and unmeasured characteristics. Allows the use of placebos and blinding.	May not be ethical or practical to randomize.
Waiting-list control (randomized)	All the advantages of randomized controls. Subjects know they will receive the intervention.	Cannot blind subjects or investigators to whether the subject is receiving the intervention.
Waiting-list control (non-randomized)	Fits clinical practice (when there is limited supply people have to wait). Only people eligible for the intervention and desirous of it will be included.	Same as randomized waiting list plus people who receive the intervention right away may be different from those waiting for it.
Concurrent control, enrolled in study	Controls do not need to receive the intervention, which may make the study easier and cheaper	Subjects who receive the intervention may be different from those who don't. Subjects may not feel motivated to participate in a study for which they derive no benefit.
Concurrent control, passively followed (e.g., medical record review)	No effort required by controls.	Subjects who receive the intervention may be different from those who don't. With passive follow-up, may lose track of subjects and not know what happened to them.
Historic control	Data may have already been collected.	Subjects who receive the intervention may be different from those who don't. Temporal changes add another source of bias.

has received it. For example, Stein and colleagues conducted a randomized study of cognitive behavioral treatment for students who reported exposure to violence and had clinical symptoms of posttraumatic stress disorder (PTSD).[2] Given that all the prospective subjects had PTSD it would be hard to not offer them treatment. Therefore, the investigators randomized subjects to the intervention or to a waiting-list group. The investigators found that students who received the intervention had significantly fewer symptoms of PTSD, less depression, and better psychosocial function than those in the waiting-list group. After the waiting-list controls received the same intervention, the two groups were similar with respect to all three measures.[3] Unfortunately, use of waiting-list controls does not allow for blinding or placebos.

[2] Stein, B. D., Jaycox, L. H., Kataoka, S. H., *et al.* "A mental health intervention for schoolchildren exposed to violence: a randomized controlled trial." *JAMA* **290** (2003): 603–11.

[3] If instead of randomizing subjects to an intervention versus waiting-list control, you randomize them to one of two different interventions, and then switch them to the other intervention after a wash-out period, you are performing a crossover design. For more see: Katz, M. H. *Study Design and Statistical Analysis: A Practical Guide for Clinicians.* Cambridge: Cambridge University Press, 2006: pp. 18–19.

At times it may not be possible to randomize subjects to be in a waiting-list group (e.g., government-sponsored services). However, if there is enough room only for a certain number of subjects to receive the intervention at any one time (e.g., an after-school program for children) subjects placed on the waiting list may be willing to be observed as part of an evaluation of the intervention.

For example, studies of the effectiveness of organ transplantation often compare individuals who receive a transplant to those who are on a waiting list for a transplant. Venstrom and colleagues used a transplant waiting list to assess the effectiveness of pancreas transplantation in patients with diabetes and preserved kidney function.[4] Using a time-dependent covariate (see Section 9.1), they demonstrated that persons receiving a solitary pancreas transplant had higher mortality (RR = 1.57; 95% CI 0.98–2.53) than persons who were waiting for a solitary pancreas transplant.

> Subjects who receive an intervention right away may be different than those left waiting.

The potential bias when using waiting-list controls that are not randomized is the possibility that persons who receive the intervention are different than those who do not. In the case of the pancreas transplantation study, those who received a pancreas transplant and those left on the waiting list were indistinguishable with respect to a number of prognostic factors including age, sex, and comorbid illness. But non-white patients were less likely to receive transplants than white patients. Although it is possible to statistically adjust for baseline differences using multivariable analysis (Chapter 7), in the absence of randomization we can never exclude the possibility that our results are biased by unmeasured characteristics.

> Patients drawn from a waiting list are by definition eligible for the intervention and desirous of it.

On the other hand, even when a waiting list is nonrandomized, using patients from a waiting list has an advantage over other nonrandomized controls. Specifically, patients drawn from a waiting list are by definition eligible for the intervention and desirous of it. Returning to the example of pancreas transplant, there are patients with a similar need for pancreas transplant who would not be eligible for transplant (e.g., actively drinking) or do not want a transplant. A control group drawn from administrative records of patients with diabetes and preserved kidney function would include such persons, but such a group would not necessarily be comparable to those patients receiving transplants.

When waiting-list controls are not possible the next best alternative is to identify a group of subjects who are willing to be observed concurrently. Unfortunately, identifying concurrent controls can be a challenge for several reasons.

---

[4] Venstrom, J. M., McBride, M. A., Rother, K. I., Hirshberg, B., Orchard, T. J., and Harlan, D. M. "Survival after pancreas transplantion in patients with diabetes and preserved kidney function." *JAMA* **290** (2003): 2817–23.

First, if they are not receiving any intervention, it may be hard to motivate subjects to participate, especially if they must devote a lot of energy to the study (e.g., completing complicated interviews or questionnaires, obtaining laboratory tests, etc.). This problem can sometimes be resolved by financially compensating subjects for their time with a stipend or by appealing to the desire to help others by advancing science.

What is harder to deal with is the likelihood that the subjects will inherently be different from those who agree to receive the intervention. In some cases, measuring the control and intervention subjects before the intervention helps to establish a baseline that can be used to adjust for baseline differences. Also, a variety of multivariable techniques can be used to adjust for baseline differences, but none of these techniques can completely eliminate bias.

An advantage of concurrent controls is that they may be less expensive than waiting-list controls if the intervention is expensive to conduct.

> Use of passively observed controls requires having an available record, such as a medical record or registry.

The challenges of concurrent controls may be less if they can be passively observed through review of a record, such as a medical record. For example, Two Feathers and colleagues evaluated a lifestyle intervention for African-Americans and Latinos with type 2 diabetes.[5] In designing the intervention the investigators worked closely with the affected community. Because of historic distrust of research, it was decided to perform the study without a randomized control group. Instead they evaluated the efficacy of the intervention by comparing glycosylated hemoglobin (Hb_{a1c}) values of participants to the values abstracted from a random sample of diabetics receiving care in the same health system. This design was possible because Hb_{a1c} assessments are uniformly ordered for diabetic patients. However, they did not have a control group for the other outcomes of their study (dietary knowledge, following a healthy eating plan, vegetable consumption). For these outcomes the investigators used a one-group pre-intervention versus post-intervention design.

Historical controls are likely to be different from your intervention subjects both because they are not part of the intervention group and because of temporal changes (even if their characteristics are exactly the same as the intervention group they were living in an earlier period). On the other hand, historic controls have one potential advantage. If a group is observed prior to an intervention being available, they could not have received the intervention. Therefore, there is less confounding due to willingness or ability to receive the intervention (there is still some confounding because were the intervention offered some of the historical controls may have said no).

[5] Two Feathers, J., Kieffer, E. C., Palmisano, G., *et al.* "Racial and ethnic approaches to community health (Reach) Detroit partnership: improving diabetes-related outcomes among African-American and Latino adults." *Am. J. Public Health* **95** (2005): 1552–60.

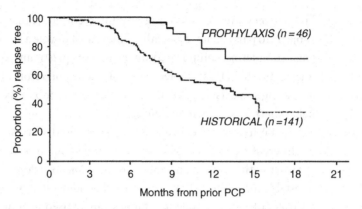

Figure 3.1

Time to PCP pneumonia among patients receiving inhaled pentamadine (prophylaxis) compared to historic controls. Reprinted from Golden, J.A., *et al.* "Prevention of *Pneumocystis carinii* pneumonia by inhaled pentamadine." *Lancet* (1989): 654–7, with permission from Elsevier.

> Historic controls are the weakest of controls.

For example, Golden and colleagues used historic controls to evaluate the effectiveness of inhaled pentamadine in preventing *Pneumocystis carinii* (*jiroveci*) pneumonia (PCP) in patients with AIDS and a prior episode of PCP.[6] At the time (1987), there were no other drugs licensed to prevent PCP and in the absence of treatment subjects had a very high risk of developing a second episode. Because recurrent PCP had a high case-fatality rate it was felt that it was unethical to have a placebo control group. Instead the authors demonstrated that subjects who received inhaled pentamadine had a much lower risk of developing a second episode than patients with a prior episode of PCP who had been diagnosed prior to the availability of inhaled pentamadine (Figure 3.1). Although historic controls are generally the weakest controls, this study helped to establish inhaled pentamadine as an effective method of prophylaxis.

3.4 How do I collect data and choose a control group for an intervention that I did not develop?

> Laws and other governmental initiatives are often launched without an evaluation plan.

Ideally, all interventions would be developed with an evaluation plan that included collecting data points prior to, during, and after the intervention as well as identifying an appropriate control group.

Unfortunately, many times an intervention will be launched without an evaluation plan. This is true of many laws, regulations, and other

---

[6] Golden, J. A., Chernoff, D., Hollander, H., Feigal, D., and Conte, J. E. "Prevention of *Pneumocystis carinii* pneumonia by inhaled pentamadine." *Lancet* (1989): 654–7.

governmental initiatives, which are often passed on the assumption that they will be beneficial.

Although challenging, evaluating interventions for which no evaluation was planned can be fruitful. For example, many of the smoking bans (e.g., no sales of tobacco to youth, no smoking in restaurants) were implemented locally, found to be effective, and were then instituted in other localities.

Even if you have not developed an intervention, if you have been closely following the development of a law or practice you may be able to launch a data collection before the intervention. More often investigators need to be creative to identify existing data and controls that can be used to evaluate interventions. Several potential sources of data and/or comparison groups are shown in Table 3.3 along with examples of intervention studies that have made use of these sources.

With the advent of electronic medical records, patient cohorts increasingly serve as a rich source of observations prior to and following an intervention as well as a source of controls. For example, the Veterans Affairs medical centers in the United States have an extensive patient database. Concato and colleagues used it to evaluate the effectiveness of screening for prostate cancer.[7] They identified 71 661 men, 50 years and older, who had an ambulatory visit to any of 10 Veterans Affairs medical Centers in New England between 1989 and 1990 and who did not have a diagnosis of prostate cancer before 1991. From this group they identified 501 men diagnosed with prostate cancer between 1991 and 1995 who died by 1999. From that same cohort they identified 501 controls who did not have prostate cancer and who matched the cases on age and site of diagnosis.

After adjustment for race and comorbidity, the investigators found that screening for prostate cancer was unassociated with mortality (OR = 1.08; 95% CI 0.71–1.64; $P = 0.72$); in other words, screening did not appear to decrease mortality. Note that at the time this study was conducted it would not have been considered ethical to randomize men to prostate screening or not because of the presumption that prostate screening saved lives.

A limitation of patient records as a data source for assessing interventions is that the records (whether electronic or paper) may not have all of the data that you need. Also subjects may be lost to follow-up without any indication of what happened to them.

Missing data and losses of subjects to follow-up are less common with ongoing research cohorts than with cohorts derived from patient records because

> Electronic patient records provide a rich source of data and controls.

> Check to see if there are any ongoing research cohorts that can be used to assess the intervention you are interested in.

[7] Concato, J., Wells, C. K., and Horwitz, R. I., *et al.* "The effectiveness of screening for prostate cancer: a nested case-control study." *Arch. Intern. Med.* **166** (2006): 38–43.

Table 3.3. Potential sources of existing data with examples of evaluations of interventions.

Source of prior observations	Example
Electronic medical records	The effectiveness of prostate screening on mortality among patients seen at one of 10 Veterans Affairs medical centers.[a]
Ongoing research cohort	The impact of postmenopausal hormone use was assessed among participants of the Nurses' Health Study.[b]
Periodic surveys	The effect of Medicaid managed care on the access to care of uninsured persons was assessed by comparing responses over time to questions from the National Health Interview Survey.[c]
Administrative databases	The impact of graduated driver licensing on car crashes among 16-year-old drivers was assessed using 3 years of crash data from Michigan State Police records.[d]
Insurance or pharmacy databases	The effect of prior authorization on decreasing the use of long-acting oxycodone was studied by comparing Medicaid prescription drug records of states with prior authorization requirements to those states that did not have such requirements.[e]
Disease or procedure databases	Drug-eluting stents were compared to coronary artery bypass grafting by identifying patients from two registries: Cardiac Surgery Reporting System and Percutaneous Coronary Intervention Reporting System of New York.[f]
Birth and death registries	The role of national health insurance in improving life expectancy was assessed using population and death registries in Taiwan.[g]

[a] Concato, J., Wells, C. K., and Horwitz, R. I., *et al.* "The effectiveness of screening for prostate cancer: a nested case-control study." *Arch. Intern. Med.* **166** (2006): 38–43.

[b] Grodstein, F., Martinez, M. E., Platz, E., *et al.* "Postmenopausal hormone use and risk for colorectal cancer and adenoma." *Ann. Intern. Med.* **128** (1998): 705–12.

[c] Haberer, J. E., Garrett, B., and Baker, L. C. "Does Medicaid managed care affect access to care for the uninsured?" *Health Affairs* **24** (2005): 1095–1105.

[d] Shope, J. T., Molnar, L. J., Elliott, M. R., and Waller, P. F. "Graduated driver licensing in Michigan: early impact on motor vehicle crashes among 16-year-old drivers." *JAMA* **286** (2001): 1593–8.

[e] Morden, N. E., Zerzan, J., Rue, T. C., *et al.* "Medicaid prior authorization and controlled-release oxycodone." *Med. Care* **16** (2008): 573–80.

[f] Hannan, E. L., Wu, C., Walford, G., *et al.* "Drug-eluting stents vs. coronary-artery bypass grafting in multivessel coronary artery disease." *N. Engl. J. Med.* **358** (2008): 331–41.

[g] Wen, C. P., Tsai, S. P., and Chung W.-S. I. "A 10-year experience with universal health insurance in Taiwan: measuring changes in health and health disparity." *Ann. Intern. Med.* **148** (2008): 258–67.

Nested case controls are a particularly time- and cost-efficient method of evaluating an intervention.

subjects are asked to make regular visits and complete standard forms, and investigators make active efforts to stay in contact with study members. For example, one of the largest and most successful cohort studies is the Nurses' Health Study. Grodstein assessed the effect of postmenopausal hormone use on the risk of colorectal cancer.[8] The investigators took advantage of self-reported data on hormone use and colorectal cancer from biennial questionnaires completed over a 14-year period among 59 002 women. After exclusion of women who reported screening sigmoidoscopy (to avoid bias due to more intensive screening among hormone users), there was a decreased risk of colorectal cancer among current hormone users (RR = 0.64; 95% CI 0.49–0.82). Nested case-control studies such as this one are particularly efficient in terms of time and cost since the data are already collected and usually in a format that makes analysis easy.

Periodic surveys repeatedly ask the same set of questions.

Periodic surveys ask the same questions each time of a sample of a population; this allows comparisons of answers prior to and after the implementation of an intervention. For example, the National Health and Nutrition Examination Survey (NHANES) interviews and performs physical examinations on a representative sample of 5000 Americans each year.

Periodic surveys can also be used to assemble a comparison group. For example, the change in an outcome before and after an intervention performed in one state can be compared to changes in the outcome at the same time points in another state where the intervention was not performed.

Municipal administrative databases are a rich and often overlooked source of data.

Municipalities have administrative databases that are a rich and often overlooked source of data. They exist on local, state, and federal levels. Examples of useful municipal databases include reports of traffic accidents, police records, jail/prison records, drug-overdose records, suicide records, medical examiner records, and supplemental income records.

Health services research has exploded with the availability of insurance and pharmacy databases. The most useful of these databases are those that include all persons in a particular group and/or all of the care that those persons receive. For example, Medicare databases include virtually all persons in the United States over 65 years and all of the hospital care they receive regardless of what hospital they were admitted to. Medicaid records (a public insurance program for low-income persons in the United States) can be used to compare policies that vary from state to state. Private health insurance providers have data sets that include all of the care that their members have received. Countries that

[8] Grodstein, F., Martinez, M. E., Platz, E., *et al.* "Postmenopausal hormone use and risk for colorectal cancer and adenoma." *Ann. Intern. Med.* **128** (1998): 705–12.

have a universal insurance system have claims for the entire country for all of the care their residents receive.

Disease- or intervention-specific databases can be particularly helpful when you need more information than would typically be available in insurance records. For example, insurance records can be effective in identifying people with certain diseases (usually through International Classification of Diseases (ICD) codes) and/or people who received certain procedures. But they do not generally include information about when the person developed the disease or, in the case of procedures, details about them (e.g., how long the patient waited for the procedure, complications associated with the procedure).

Birth and death registries are essential for calculating mortality and life expectancy. Birth registries often have additional data about perinatal outcomes such as birth weight and death registries generally include cause of death, as well as factors contributing to death.

To evaluate some interventions it may be necessary to link several of the databases listed in Table 3.3. For example, Lipscombe and colleagues sought to determine whether the use of thiazolidinediones (TZD) in diabetics was associated with cardiovascular disease.[9] To do so they linked a prescription record database (use of hypoglycemic agents), an ambulatory care database (emergency room records), a hospital database (hospital admission records), a health insurance plan database (physician records), a vital status database (demographics and mortality), and a disease-specific database (diabetes records). They found that use of TZD treatment was associated with increased risk of congestive heart failure, acute myocardial infarction, and death.

All of the databases listed in Table 3.3 can be used to identify controls. However, if you review the different types of controls listed in Table 3.2 you realize that randomized controls will rarely be an option. An exception would be a government intervention that was distributed on a random basis; for example, affordable housing is often distributed based on a lottery of persons who meet the eligibility criteria and submit their application within a window period. A registry of persons who did and did not receive housing by a particular date based on randomization would provide the basis for a very robust evaluation of a housing initiative.

More commonly, nonrandomized controls will be used (such as in the studies of prostate and colon cancer discussed above). For studies of laws or institutional practices, samples of persons from other geographic areas of a town, city, state, or country are a good source of controls.

---

[9] Lipscombe, L. L., Gomes, T., Levesque, L. E., Hux, J. E., Juurlink, D. N., and Alter, D. A. "Thiazolidinediones and cardiovascular outcomes in older patients with diabetes." *JAMA* **298** (2007): 2634–43.

Evaluations of existing interventions can be very inexpensive.

I hope that I have convinced you that you can successfully perform an evaluation of an intervention for which no evaluation was planned. Now let me mention two advantages of this type of study. First, they are often relatively inexpensive to perform because you do not have to pay for the intervention. Second, to the extent that the intervention has been widely implemented, a negative study (one that shows no impact of the intervention) has as much impact as a positive study. Why? Because by identifying an existing implementation that is not working, you may save costs for the system by eliminating an ineffective intervention. You also may spur development of new methods where there was previously complacency due to the belief that the existing intervention worked. We will take up the issue of studies with negative results again in Section 9.8.

3.5 What outcomes of an intervention should I assess?

It is common to hear policy and legislative leaders speak of the need to evaluate a particular program to find out whether it works. But if you asked them what would convince them that the program was a success you may be surprised at the variety of responses.

I was meeting with a group of stakeholders – health, business, civic, and union leaders – to develop a universal health access program for my county. Throughout the process many participants spoke of the importance of evaluating whether the program worked. At one of the sessions, I asked them what outcome, five years in the future, would make them believe that the program had worked. Each one had a different answer: more people coming forward for care, higher satisfaction with care, more preventive care, fewer emergency department visits, improved health status, lower costs. Each of these outcomes is potentially important, but each requires a somewhat different approach.

The most important step in planning an evaluation is to decide what outcome(s) you are going to assess.

Therefore, the most important step in planning an evaluation of a program is to decide what outcome(s) you are going to assess. In some cases, the ideal outcome may not be feasible. For example, for many medical interventions increasing lifespan is the most important outcome, but using death as a study outcome may not be feasible if the study period is relatively short.

A proximal marker is predictive of a particular outcome but occurs earlier and therefore results in more study outcomes in shorter follow-up times.

In situations where the outcome of interest takes a long time to occur, you may need to use a proximal marker. A proximal marker is highly predictive of the outcome you wish to study but occurs earlier and therefore results in more outcomes in shorter follow-up times. For example, glycosylated hemoglobin (Hb_{a1c}) is a marker of diabetes control that predicts complications of diabetes.

3.6 Why measure the exposure of subjects to an intervention?

Those among you who have not yet performed an intervention trial may assume that people who participate in a study and are assigned to an intervention receive it and those not assigned to an intervention do not. If only this were the case trial results would be so much easier to interpret! More commonly, some subjects in the intervention group don't receive the intervention and some in the control group do. It is critical to the interpretation of the results of a study to measure exposure to the intervention. Why?

> Measure exposure to your intervention.

Let's start with the case of an intervention that appears to work. Showing that people who were assigned to the intervention group actually received the intervention (and those who were not assigned to the intervention did not receive it) strengthens the validity of the study.

> Measure the intensity of the exposure.

Exposure should be measured in terms of the intensity of the exposure (e.g., percent of doses taken, number of visits made, etc.) not just as whether the intervention was received – yes or no. In this way you may test for dose–response relationships (persons who receive a more intense exposure to the intervention should show greater changes). Dose–response relationships strengthen causal inference – the assumption that the intervention produces the demonstrated result.

Alternatively, if most people in the intervention group had no or minimal exposure to the intervention, then the apparent effect of the intervention might be due to some other factor.

In the case of an intervention that does not appear to work, it is important to determine whether it didn't work because the intervention is ineffective, or because the participants were not sufficiently exposed to the intervention, or because too many people in the control group were exposed to the intervention. Understanding the reason that an intervention did not work is critical to the design of future studies.

For example, O'Loughlin and colleagues evaluated a community-based cardiovascular program performed in a low-income community of Montreal, Quebec.[10] A nearby community served as the control. At the three-year follow-up there were no declines in smoking or in eating high-fat foods in either the intervention or the control community; physical inactivity actually increased in both communities. However, participation in the program was very low. Participation in the walking club, workshops in healthy eating and weight reduction, videos, and contests were each less than 1.5% of the population.

---

[10] O'Loughlin, J. L., Paradis, G., Gray-Donald, K., and Renaud, L. "The impact of a community-based heart disease prevention program in a low-income, inner-city neighborhood." *Am. J. Public Health* **89** (1999); 1819–26.

Given this level of participation, it would not be realistic to expect the intervention to have worked.

It is also not realistic to expect the intervention group to do better than the control group if a lot of the control patients are exposed to the intervention. For example, in a randomized study of an educational intervention to decrease hospital-wide infections (e.g., increased hand-washing, avoiding inappropriate antibiotic use), doctors randomized to no intervention may change their behavior, just due to observing their colleagues. (I'm using the example of hospital-wide infections to help you remember how contamination can occur in a research setting!) To decrease contamination, studies of observable behavior often perform randomization by group, such as by hospital or by school (Section 4.5).

> Contamination occurs when members of the control group are exposed to the intervention.

3.7 Should I use a longitudinal cohort or a serial cross-sectional design?

As discussed in Section 1.2.A, there are two ways of performing pre-intervention versus post-intervention assessments: assessing the same people over time (longitudinal cohort) and serial (repeated) sampling from the same population (serial cross-sectional design). The two designs have different advantages and disadvantages (Table 3.4).

The major advantage of longitudinal studies (the more commonly used design) is that each person can serve as his or her own control. For example, if the outcome of interest is weight loss at 6 months, weight at baseline can serve as the starting point for each subject. This minimizes the importance of differences in baseline weight between subjects in the different groups.

Another advantage of longitudinal studies is that all or most of the subjects in the intervention group will have received the intervention, making it easier to demonstrate an effect of the intervention. This is not true when you perform repeated cross-sectional samples of a community. Depending on how extensively the intervention has been disseminated in the population, you may find a relatively small proportion of persons who have actually been exposed to it.

However, longitudinal cohort studies also have problems when used to evaluate interventions. If you ask subjects the same questions repeatedly, your questioning is likely to affect their answers. In particular, in longitudinal studies participants generally interact repeatedly with study staff and often develop strong loyalty to them – a good thing when you need people to attend repeated visits. However, the bond between subjects and study personnel can be detrimental if participants respond to questions the way they believe the investigators want them to (rather than telling the truth). (If you have any doubts about this, how honest were you the last time your dentist asked you how often you flossed your teeth?)

Table 3.4. Comparison of longitudinal cohort and serial cross-sectional designs.

Design	Advantages	Disadvantages
Longitudinal cohort	Greater power because subjects serve as their own control. Easier to sample persons who have actually received the intervention.	Expensive to track people over time. Observing individuals repeatedly in a trial may slant their answers (e.g., socially desirable responses). Subjects can be lost to follow-up.
Serial cross-sectional	Subject responses are less likely to be influenced by study participation. No requirement to follow subjects over time. No subjects are lost to follow-up. Best model for demonstrating changes in a population. Only method that can be used to study changes in practice patterns.	Decreased power due to having to account for variance between subjects. May have low exposure to the intervention among subjects.

> Socially desirable responses occur when subjects tell you what you want to hear.

Social desirability responses can be particularly an issue with intervention trials because subjects will know the goal of the study is to change their behavior and they will not want to displease the study staff by admitting to behavior they know is wrong (e.g., admitting to drug use when in a study of drug treatment).

The best way to avoid the problem of social desirability in responses is to have an objective marker of behavior (e.g., saliva test for cigarette smoking). However, this is not always possible. With serial cross-sectional studies subjects have not been asked the same question repeatedly and have not interacted extensively with study staff; therefore their answers are less likely to be influenced by their participation in the study.

> Use serial cross-sectional designs to demonstrate changes in a population.

Besides being less likely to elicit socially desirable responses, serial cross-sectional designs are superior when you are trying to demonstrate that an intervention has affected a whole community. For example, the Minnesota Heart Health Program was a large community intervention involving 400 000 persons in six communities.[11] The goal of the intervention was to reduce morbidity and mortality from cardiovascular disease. Three communities received individual, group, and community-level programming designed to decrease blood pressure, improve healthy eating, decrease smoking, and increase activity. The program was evaluated by conducting cross-sectional surveys of 300–500 persons in each community seven to eight times over a

[11] Luepker, R. V., Murray, D. M., Jacobs, D. R., *et al.* "Community education for cardiovascular disease prevention: risk factor changes in the Minnesota Heart Health Program." *Am. J. Public Health* **84** (1994): 1383–93.

decade. A serial cross-sectional design made sense because the goal was to change the behavior of the entire community, not just persons enrolled in an intervention.

> Studies of changes in medical practice usually require serial cross-sectional designs.

To evaluate changes in medical practice, in most cases you will have no choice but to use serial cross-sections. To see why look back at Table 1.2. The data are from a study of whether providing hospitals with confidential information on their performance improves their care of patients having coronary artery bypass grafting (CABG). The investigators looked at four measures of quality of CABG. A longitudinal study would not work because once patients have had their surgery, it's not possible to evaluate whether surgery techniques improved. (Even if a patient had a repeat CABG it would not be the same. Patients who require a repeat surgery are different than first-comers – the outcome of the first surgery would affect the second one.) Instead, you must look at serial cross-sections of cardiac patients to see whether surgery practice improved.

> Serial cross-sectional studies may be cheaper to conduct than longitudinal cohort studies.

Serial cross-sectional studies may be cheaper than longitudinal cohort studies because there is no need to stay in contact with subjects. Even with extensive follow-up some subjects will be lost to follow-up in longitudinal cohort studies; this cannot occur with serial cross-sectional studies.

Because they have different advantages and disadvantages, investigators of population-level interventions may perform both. In fact, the Minnesota Heart Health Program supplemented the cross-sectional samples by taking a sample of participants from the pre-intervention cross-sectional surveys and following them over time (longitudinal cohort). Results were similar: with both the cross-sectional samples and the cohort sample, the intervention did not produce substantially greater improvements in cardiac risk factors than those seen in the comparison groups.

Serial cross-sectional studies require a different statistical approach than longitudinal studies. These are covered in Sections 6.3 and 6.5, respectively.

3.8 How do I develop measurement instruments?

The type of measurement instruments you will need to develop will depend on what you are studying and how you will be collecting your data (e.g., questionnaires, interviews, observations, etc.). This is beyond the scope of this book.[12]

---

[12] For a good introduction to these issues see Kelsy, J. L., Whittemore, A. S., Evans, A. S., and Thompson, W. D. *Methods in Observational Epidemiology* (2nd edition). Oxford: Oxford University Press, 1996: pp. 364–412.

To perform your analysis you will also need to manage your data (enter it, clean it, recode, transform, and derive variables) and export it into a software package that can perform the needed analyses.[13]

3.9 How do I state the hypothesis of an intervention study?

Every intervention study should have a hypothesis – what it is you are trying to prove. To facilitate statistical testing, the hypothesis should be stated in the null form. The null hypotheses for the three major questions of intervention studies (Section 1.2) are:

1 There is no change between the pre-intervention and the post-intervention assessment.
2 The change between the pre-intervention and the post-intervention assessment is no greater in the intervention group than the change in the comparison group.
3 The outcome for the intervention group is no different from that of the comparison group.

We use statistics to determine the probability that the null hypothesis is correct. If the probability is very low, we consider the alternative hypothesis: that the intervention is associated with a significant change. The three null hypotheses can be restated as alternative hypotheses, as follows:

1 There is a change between the pre-intervention and the post-intervention assessment.
2 The change between the pre-intervention and the post-intervention assessment in the intervention group is greater/less than the change in the comparison group.
3 The outcome for the intervention group is different than that of the comparison group.

Note that the alternative hypothesis is stated in a neutral direction (e.g., alternative hypothesis #1 doesn't say whether the change between the pre-intervention and the post-intervention assessment is up or down). This is referred to as a two-sided hypothesis.

Even though the alternative hypothesis is best stated in a neutral way, you can have an opinion; for example, you may believe that the intervention group will do better than the non-intervention group. In fact, if you didn't have an

> Alternative hypotheses should be stated in a neutral direction.

[13] Katz, M. H. *Study Design and Statistical Analysis: A Practical Guide for Clinicians.* Cambridge: Cambridge University Press, 2006: pp. 38–51.

opinion, in many cases, you wouldn't do the study. Still, it is generally best to state and test the hypothesis in a neutral way.

In rare cases it may be appropriate to state and test a one-sided alternative hypothesis. The rationale for stating a one-sided alternative hypothesis is that only one side of the hypothesis is possible or of interest. For example, Nadelman and colleagues studied the efficacy of doxycycline in preventing Lyme disease in an area where the disease was hyperendemic.[14] Subjects who had removed an attached *I. scapularis* tick from their body within the prior 72 hours were randomized to either a single dose of doxycycline or placebo. It is very unlikely that a single dose of doxycycline could increase the risk of developing Lyme disease and the investigators therefore considered their hypothesis to be one-sided.

The benefit of testing a one-sided hypothesis is that it is easier to detect a statistical association: a smaller sample size is required to demonstrate a given effect size. For example, a given effect size and sample size that results in a *P* value of 0.08 with a two-sided test (hypotheses have "sides" and tests have "tails"), would have a *P* value of 0.04 with a one-sided test. Given the slavish attention paid to the arbitrary cut-off of 0.05, you can see why some investigators prefer a one-tailed test.

The problem with one-sided hypotheses is being certain that only one direction of the alternative hypothesis is possible. For example, Pletcher and colleagues developed an intervention to improve treatment of alcohol withdrawal in hospitalized patients.[15] The intervention was to promulgate quality guidelines for the care of patients in their hospital based on the published literature and recommendations of a prominent specialty society. The problem was when they evaluated the impact of the new guidelines using a pre-intervention versus post-intervention design (since this was a typical hospital quality improvement program no control group was used), they found a significant increase of in-hospital deaths after the guidelines were implemented.

> **TIP**
> Use two-tailed tests.

Therefore, even if one side of the hypothesis seems very unlikely, you will do better to use a two-tailed test. Two-sided hypotheses and tests are more rigorous and they are what most journal editors expect.

Going back to the doxycycline treatment example, even though the authors specified a single-sided hypothesis, they ultimately performed a two-tailed test. They found that erythema migrans (rash diagnostic of Lyme disease) developed at the site of the tick bite in 8 of the 247 subjects who received placebo

[14] Nadelman, R. B., Nowakowski, J., Fish, D., *et al.* "Prophylaxis with single-dose doxycycline for the prevention of Lyme disease after an ixodes scapularis tick bite." *N. Engl. J. Med.* **345** (2001): 79–84.

[15] Pletcher, M. J., Fernandez, A., May, T. A., *et al.* "Unintended consequences of a quality improvement program designed to improve treatment of alcohol withdrawal in hospitalized patients." *Jt. Comm. J. Qual. Patient Saf.* **31** (2005): 148–157.

compared to 1 of the 235 subjects in the doxycycline group ($P < 0.04$). Because the two-tailed test was under the statistical threshold of $P = 0.05$ the decision to use a two-tailed test had no impact on whether the result was considered statistically significant. Would they have reported their results in the same way if their two-tailed P value had been $P = 0.06$? I would hope so, but I know for sure that whether the results were P equals 0.06 or equals 0.04, I would take doxycycline following an *I. scapularis* tick bite.

3.10 Can an intervention study have more than one hypothesis?

Multiple outcomes can strengthen an intervention study.

Yes. It is often better to specify more than one hypothesis (to assess whether the intervention is associated with more than one outcome). This can strengthen a study by demonstrating that the intervention has multiple positive effects. For example, an exercise intervention might decrease weight, improve muscle mass, decrease blood pressure, decrease fasting blood glucose, and improve mood.

Demonstrating that an intervention affects multiple outcomes on a causal pathway also increases the validity of your results. For example, it would be more believable that an intervention decreases diabetic retinopathy if it also decreases fasting blood glucose.

However, when you test for multiple differences between groups, the likelihood increases that at least one of these comparisons will be statistically significant. In fact, if you compare an intervention to a placebo on 20 different outcomes you would expect that one of the comparisons would be significant at the $P < 0.05$ threshold by chance alone.

To avoid this problem, distinguish the primary outcome from the secondary outcomes in the analysis plan. You will then need to adjust your significance level for the multiple comparisons. Methods for adjustment for multiple comparisons are discussed in Section 9.3.

3.11 Why should I have an analysis plan?

Write an analysis plan prior to unblinding group assignment and/or analyzing your data.

Every study should have an analysis plan. In the case of a randomized study it should be written prior to randomizing subjects (ideally), but definitely prior to unblinding group assignment and/or performing any data analysis. In the case of a nonrandomized intervention, it should be written prior to data collection (ideally), but definitely prior to data analysis.

An analysis plan details how the data will be analyzed once they are collected. It should include the major outcome of interest (e.g., weight loss) as well as secondary outcomes (e.g., fasting glucose level). The study hypotheses should be stated in both the null form and the alternative form (Section 3.9).

The plan should state what statistics will be used to test the hypotheses. For example: the null hypothesis is that there will be no difference in weight loss between subjects randomized to the intervention and those randomized to usual care; this will be tested by comparing the weight change in the intervention group to the weight change in the usual care group using a two-tailed *t*-test (Section 6.2). If you have multiple outcomes (Section 3.10), state how you will adjust for multiple comparisons (Section 9.3). If you are planning to do any subgroup analysis (Section 9.5) this should be described.

The analysis plan should state whether there will be any interim analyses to assess whether the study should be terminated early (Section 9.4). It should state whether the data will be analyzed using intention-to-treat, per-protocol analyses, or both (Section 4.8). It should also state how you will handle missing data (e.g., excluding missing values, imputing values) (Section 9.6).

| Pre-specifying the analysis will decrease false positive results. |

There are several reasons why it is important to write an analysis plan prior to analyzing your data. First, pre-specifying the analysis will decrease bias and prevent false positive results. To understand why, consider an extreme example. As you analyze your data, you construct a composite outcome that maximizes the apparent effectiveness of the intervention. You do this by grouping outcomes that are related to the intervention (this would lead to a type 1 error – falsely concluding that the intervention works when the null hypothesis is true).

When analyzing study data there are many decisions to be made along the way (how to code a variable, how to deal with missing data) and if each of these decisions is not decided ahead, the natural tendency will be to choose the method that produces the effect you are trying to demonstrate, thus biasing your results. By pre-specifying how you will analyze your data you are protecting the integrity of your analysis.

Besides these reasons, it is not possible to conduct a sample size calculation (Section 3.12) without knowing how you will analyze your data. You will also find that considering ahead of time how you will conduct your analysis will help ensure that you collect all the data you will need to answer your question (e.g., covariates).

Finally, having a preset analysis plan should prevent the selective reporting of results (e.g., reporting only those results that supported the study hypothesis or changing outcomes midstream). Unfortunately, even an analysis plan does not always prevent investigators from straying: a study comparing published randomized reports with their study protocols found that reporting was often biased and inconsistent with the protocol; specifically 62% of trials had at least one primary outcome that was changed, introduced, or omitted.[16]

Post-hoc analyses are those that arise during the data analysis process.

Having an analysis plan should not prevent pursuing analyses that arise during the analysis. Such analyses are called post-hoc analyses and can be very valuable. However, the *P* values associated with these results substantially underestimate the likelihood that the findings are due to chance. For this reason, results from post-hoc analyses should be viewed more tentatively than those from pre-specified analyses. This is especially true if the analysis is suggested by your data analysis (as opposed to a new question that arose after the pre-analysis plan was formulated).

The *P* values associated with post-hoc analyses substantially underestimate the likelihood that the findings are due to chance.

3.12 How do I calculate sample size for an intervention study?

Calculation of sample size for intervention studies is no different mathematically than the calculation of sample size for other types of studies. The number of subjects needed depends on the estimated size of the effect of the intervention, the number of groups studied, the type of outcome measure (e.g., interval, ordinal), the variability of the measurements (e.g., standard error), the number of covariates in the model (assuming multivariable analysis will be performed), the duration of follow-up (for studies of time), and the number of subjects lost to follow-up.

Because it is not mathematically different, I will not review the methods, but instead direct you to the references, which include free software for calculating sample size.[17]

Power your study so that you can rule out a meaningful effect if there is none.

What is critically important with intervention studies is to ensure that the study is sufficiently powered to rule out an intervention effect. Otherwise, if the intervention does not work you will not know whether the reason was that the intervention was ineffective or that the study was underpowered. This is unfair to the subjects who have donated their time, and does not further science.[18]

---

[16] Chan, A. W., Hrobjartsson, A., Haahr, M. T., Gotzsche, P. C., and Altman, D. G. "Empirical evidence for selective reporting of outcomes in randomized trials: comparison of protocols to published articles." *JAMA* **291** (2004): 2457–65.

[17] For a free software program for calculating sample size go to www.openepi.com. It calculates sample size for proportions and means for unmatched case-control and cohort studies including trials. For more complicated designs including matched case-control, linear regression, and survival analysis go to: www.mc.vanderbilt.edu/prevmed/ps (also free). For a detailed discussion on sample size see Friedman, L. M., Furberg, C. D., and DeMets, D. L. *Fundamentals of Clinical Trials* (3rd edition). New York: Springer, 1999: pp. 94–129. For a simpler version see: Katz, M. H. *Study Design and Statistical Analysis: A Practical Guide for Clinicians.* Cambridge: Cambridge University Press: 1996: pp. 127–40.

[18] Halpern, S. D., Karlawish J. H. T., and Berlin, J. A. "The continuing unethical conduct of underpowered clinical trials." *JAMA* **288** (2002): 358–62.

I will take up this subject again later in the section on publishing negative studies (Section 9.8).

3.13 How do I obtain an institutional review board (IRB) review for a study?

All studies involving human subjects require a review by an institutional review board (IRB). These boards, also known as human subjects committees, review the goals and procedures of your study to be certain that the rights of human subjects are protected.

> Informed consent is needed unless risks to individuals are very minimal or consent is impossible to obtain.

A key determination is whether the investigators must obtain informed consent of the subjects and how the informed consent will be obtained (e.g., signed, verbal assent). The usual reason for not requiring informed consent is that the risk to the individual is very minimal (e.g., medical record review) or consent is impossible (e.g., a study of the best method to resuscitate patients found down in the field).

Many funders require IRB approval prior to even funding a study. Most journals will not publish studies that have not been appropriately reviewed by an IRB.

As implied by the name, IRBs are usually associated with an institution such as a university or governmental entity. The members are drawn from a variety of disciplines and should ideally include clinicians, ethicists, researchers, lawyers, and research subjects or their advocates.

Although all studies involving human subjects should be reviewed by an IRB, an IRB may make the decision to grant the study an exemption or waiver, meaning it does not require the approval process of the committee. Waivers are granted to studies that have no or little potential for harm of human subjects, such as a hospital quality improvement program, an analysis of an administrative database with no identifiers, a descriptive review of a novel clinical program where all the data were collected as part of the clinical work, or a research study conducted as part of governmental public health efforts (e.g., a disease-outbreak investigation).

To illustrate the complexity of issues concerning IRBs, informed consent, and waivers, let me tell you what happened with the study on reducing catheter-related infections by Pronovost and colleagues (Section 1.2.A). It caused a huge stir in the IRB world, played out on the pages of the *New York Times*.

Here are the basic facts.[19] Provonost and colleagues sought to implement a quality improvement project to reduce catheter-related infections in 67

---

[19] For more on this case and the practical and ethical issues it raises see Miller, F. G. and Emanuel, E. "Quality-improvement research and informed consent." *N. Engl. J. Med.* **358** (2008): 765–7; Baily, M. A. "Harming through protection?" *N. Engl. J. Med.* **358** (2008): 768–9.

Michigan hospitals. The study protocol was submitted to the IRB at Johns Hopkins University. The IRB judged that the intervention was exempt from review because it was a quality improvement program. Therefore, informed consent of patients was waived.

The Federal Office for Human Research Protections (OHRP) received a written complaint that the research was conducted without the review of an IRB and without the informed consent of the subjects. As a result of the investigation the study was voluntarily halted. The OHRP ruled that the Johns Hopkins IRB should have reviewed the study (not made it exempt) and that informed consent should have been obtained from the subjects (from both the patients and the physicians who participated in sessions on how to reduce infections).

Both parts of this decision have been hotly debated. Hospital leaders, who have been performing quality improvement efforts for decades without IRB approval or informed consent of patients, were concerned that requiring IRB review and informed consent would be onerous and discourage attempts to improve quality. To calm these protests, OHRP offered a new pathway that struck many of us in the research community as illogical. The OHRP ruled that hospitals could conduct quality improvement programs without IRB review so long as the sole aim was to improve patient care – in other words, as long as the hospital did not assess whether the practice worked! Many of us feel that it is unethical to engage in quality improvement programs without assessing whether they work. (If you have any doubt of this look back at the example of the quality improvement program for the treatment of alcohol withdrawal in Section 3.9; the quality improvement effort was associated with increased mortality.) Besides making sure that the intervention really works, isn't it unethical not to tell others what they can do to improve patient care?

Nonetheless, if you receive a research grant to do a study, and/or think there is a chance that you will publish the results of the study (two criteria that OHRP considers when deciding whether you are doing more than implementing an intervention to improve quality), submit the protocol to the IRB even if you think it should be waived. This applies to any study of human subjects (e.g., review of administrative data, descriptive review of a clinical program). They can perform an expedited review of it.

> If you receive a grant or intend to publish your research, submit your protocol to an IRB for review.

Obtaining informed consent is a much more challenging issue. It greatly complicates a study, results in some people not participating, and in the case of a quality improvement program has the complication of it being unclear what to do if the person does not want to participate. Given that the protocol of Provonost and colleagues included only interventions that were considered standard of care (e.g., hand-washing), it is unclear what the alternative to participation would be. Would you tell the patient that if he or she did not wish to be in the study then the nurse would not remind the doctor to wash his or her hands? I would hope not. I suppose you could tell them that you wouldn't include them in the recording of results.

Fortunately OHRP appears to have softened their stance; they are allowing informed consent to be waived in certain quality improvement programs. (Indeed, when the Johns Hopkins IRB reviewed the study in response to the OHRP investigation, they granted the investigators a waiver for patient consent.) By submitting your protocol for IRB review, you will learn from the experts whether or not you can waive informed consent.

The events surrounding the study of decreasing ICU infections also illustrate another important point: there can be disagreements in the interpretation of the rules governing human subject protection. If you ever conduct a multi-center trial where you are required to obtain approval of the IRB associated with each institution you will see this point played out in subtle ways. Each IRB will try to edit your consents in different ways to fit their sense of how to best obtain informed consent.

3.14 When do I need an independent data and safety monitoring committee?

If you are conducting a prospective randomized study where participants and/or their doctors do not know the treatment they are receiving (double-blinded), then you need to set up an independent data and safety monitoring committee. The committee reviews events that occur during the study that could require stopping the study or withdrawing individual patients. Unlike the investigators, the independent data and safety monitoring committee may unblind the assignment if it is for the benefit of the subjects without introducing bias into the study. If your study has pre-specified interim analyses (Section 3.11) with early stopping rules (Section 9.4), the data and safety monitoring committee should perform the analysis.

3.15 Why should I register my trial?

Publication bias favors studies with positive findings.

Trial registration is an important method of ensuring that all of the evidence on a topic is available to clinicians, consumers, and researchers. Prior to the establishment of registries, unpublished trials were hard to find. This is a problem because negative studies (those where the intervention is not found to be effective) are less likely to be published.[20] Without the ability to identify unpublished studies, reviews of prior research will probably overestimate the effectiveness of the interventions. Making it easy to find all the available studies is of even greater significance with the growing reliance on systemic reviews (meta-analyses) for making clinical and policy decisions.

Which intervention studies should be registered? According to the International Committee of Medical Journal Editors: "Any research project that prospectively assigns human subjects to intervention and comparison groups to study the cause-and-effect relationship between a medical intervention and a health outcome."[21] Both randomized and nonrandomized prospective studies should be registered. Retrospective studies, pharmokinetic studies, and phase 1 trials of toxicity do not require registration.

If I haven't convinced you of the value of registering your trial, consider this: All major journals require it! There are several available trial registries:

> All major journals require trial registration.

http://www.anzctr.org.au
http://www.clinicaltrials.gov
http://isrctn.org
http://www.trialregister.nl/trialreg/index.asp
http://www.umin.ac.jp/ctr

All these trial registries include the minimum necessary data set including information about the methods and results.

---

[20] Klassen, T. P., Wiebe, N., Russell, K., *et al.* "Abstracts of randomized controlled trials presented at the society for pediatric research meeting: an example of publication bias." *Arch. Pediatr. Adolesc. Med.* **156** (2002): 474–9.

[21] De Angelis, C., Drazen, J. M., Frizelle, F. A., *et al.* "Is this clinical trial fully registered?" A statement from the International Committee of Medical Journal Editors. www.icmje.org/clin_trialup.htm.

Randomized designs

4.1 What are randomized studies?

Random assignment is assignment by chance.

In a randomized study, subjects are assigned to each group by chance, such as by the flip of a coin. This is known as random assignment and should not be confused with random selection, which is the selection of cases from a population at random. To illustrate the difference: if you have a nonrandom sample, such as a convenience sample of patients in a clinic, you can still randomize them to different groups.

Use a computerized number generator to randomly assign subjects to study groups.

Although an unbiased coin would work perfectly well for randomizing subjects to two groups, randomization is generally performed using a computerized random number generator: you specify the number of groups you want to create and what proportion you want in each group (for example, in studies of equal allocation you would specify that you wanted half the subjects in each group), and the computer will spit out numbers that can be used to assign subjects randomly to the groups.[1]

4.2 What are the advantages of randomization?

Randomization produces groups unbiased by factors that may favor one group over the others.

The major advantage of randomization is that it produces unbiased groups; that is, because group assignment is determined randomly it cannot be influenced by factors that may otherwise confound the results of the study.

Confounders are factors that are associated with group assignment and are causally related to outcome. Because there is no relationship between potential confounders and group assignment in a randomized controlled trial, we can be confident that any differences that develop between the groups are not due to confounders (Figure 4.1).

In comparison, when assignments are not randomized, a number of factors (e.g., patient preferences, family or social group preferences, physician

---

[1] A free, easy-to-use random number generator is available at www.randomizer.org. Random numbers produced by a computer algorithm are technically not random, but pseudorandom (an insight I owe to Josephine Wolf); nonetheless, they work well for study purposes.

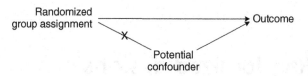

Figure 4.1

With randomized group assignment there is no relationship between potential confounders and group assignment; therefore there can be no confounding.

preferences, investigator preferences) may influence whether or not a subject takes a particular medication, follows a diet, obeys a law, etc. These factors may also be causally related to outcome (e.g., persons compliant with medications may live longer because they engage in a variety of health-promoting behaviors such as visiting the doctor regularly, following medical advice) and thereby confound the results of your study.

> Randomization tends to produce groups that are similar on baseline characteristics.

Because assignment is unbiased when randomized, randomization tends to produce groups that are comparable on baseline characteristics (i.e., each group has a similar proportion of men and women, younger and older people, healthier and sicker persons). Comparability of groups at baseline is essential to ascribing differences between the intervention group and the comparison group to the intervention, rather than to inherent characteristics of the group (e.g., healthier people are more likely to survive surgery than sicker people).

Comparability of groups is so important that the results section of almost every published intervention study begins with a "Table 1" comparing the baseline characteristics of the study groups. In the case of randomized studies, the groups are expected to be similar.

> Randomization does not guarantee that the groups will be the same on every characteristic.

Unfortunately, randomization does not guarantee that the groups will be similar on every characteristic in every randomized study. Sometimes by chance (bad luck!) randomization will produce groups that have important differences on baseline characteristics. For example, DiClemente and Wingood randomized 128 women to one of three groups: a five-session social skills HIV-prevention program; a one-session education group; or a delayed education control. Despite the randomization, at baseline women randomized to the social skills intervention were in longer-term relationships (45 months) than women in the HIV education group (21 months) and the delay control group (33 months) ($P = 0.06$). Also participants in the delayed group were more likely (83%) to be very poor (income less than $400 per month) than those in the intervention group (72%) and those in the education control (60%) ($P = 0.10$).[2]

---

[2] DiClemente, R. J. and Wingood, G. M. "A randomized controlled trial of an HIV sexual risk-reduction intervention for young African-American women." *JAMA* **274** (1995): 1271–6.

Note that neither of these baseline differences reached the conventional significance level of $P < 0.05$. However, baseline difference between study groups where the variable is associated with the outcome can be a confounder even if the difference between the groups does not reach statistical significance. Also, you can have several variables that are each a little different between the groups, with all variables favoring one group (subjects in one group are somewhat younger, somewhat less likely to be smokers, and somewhat less likely to have an underlying disease). While none of these differences may even approach statistical significance together they may result in one group being more likely to have a particular outcome regardless of the intervention.

> Baseline differences between groups can confound the results even if the differences are not statistically significant.

> Small, non-significant differences between groups on a number of different variables may still confound the results especially if the differences on the variables all favor one group.

Did the differences in the baseline characteristics of the women in the HIV-prevention study of DiClemente and Wingood invalidate the study? No. However, the differences between the groups required the investigators to adjust their analysis for income and length of current relationship using multivariable analysis.

Because even small differences in baseline characteristics can potentially bias the results of studies, investigators performing randomized studies are increasingly using multivariable analysis just as you would do to adjust for baseline differences with nonrandomized studies.

> The power of randomization is the ability to produce groups that are similar on unmeasured characteristics.

Whether or not you adjust for baseline differences, the true power of randomization is that it produces groups that are similar on **unmeasured** characteristics. This is critical because it is impossible to adjust for unmeasured or unknown characteristics. Therefore, in a nonrandomized design, even if the groups are balanced on all measured characteristics known to affect outcome, there remains a question as to whether differences that occur during the course of the study are due to the intervention or to some unknown characteristic.

A final advantage of randomization is that it ensures that the significance levels of the statistical techniques used to analyze data are valid.[3]

4.3 What are the disadvantages of randomization?

Although randomization is the best way of determining whether an intervention works, it has several disadvantages.

> Randomization cannot be used to study some interventions such as the impact of laws.

Foremost, in many cases randomization is impossible. For example, it is important to understand whether changes in laws (e.g., requirements that children be placed in car safety seats, taxes on tobacco) are having a beneficial effect. Since it is not possible to randomize people to be subject to the law other designs are needed.

---

[3] For more on this point, and a more detailed discussion of randomized controlled trials see: Friedman, L. M., Furberg, C. D., and DeMets, D. L. *Fundamentals of Clinical Trials* (3rd edition). New York: Springer, 1999: pp. 43–6.

To randomize subjects, there must be a state of equipoise, meaning that the arms of the study are believed to be equal. This does not mean that everyone believes that they are equal; in fact, a perfect situation for randomization is one where half the doctors feel treatment A is clearly superior and the other half believe that treatment B is clearly superior.

However, if one treatment is thought to be superior then it may be considered unethical to randomize people. For example, it was thought to be unethical to randomize critically ill patients to receive or not receive a pulmonary artery catheter because the catheter was thought essential to managing medications and fluids for these patients. However, when a well-done nonrandomized study showed that patients were more likely to die if they had a catheter placed,[4] enough doubt was introduced that a randomized controlled trial became possible; it showed that patients randomized to receive a pulmonary artery catheter had greater mortality,[5] and this has resulted in a substantial decrease in the use of pulmonary artery catheters.

| Randomized designs often have limited generalizability. |

Even when randomization is feasible and ethical, these designs have limited generalizability. Randomized controlled trials are conducted under strict conditions: subjects must consent themselves to be randomized; they must make frequent study visits; and they must agree to intrusive questions and often laboratory tests. Therefore, subjects who are willing to enter and remain in randomized controlled trials are different from other subjects. Also, the medical care delivered within these trials is different from the medical care delivered in normal clinical practice.

| Hawthorne effect is when the behavior of subjects changes simply due to being observed. |

Not only are the subjects in randomized controlled trials different, and treated differently, but their behavior may actually change simply due to being observed. This is referred to as the Hawthorne effect.[6] The Hawthorne effect is not unique to randomized controlled trials. However, the more intense observation in these trials compared to most observational trials makes the Hawthorne effect potentially more potent.

4.4 What are the different methods of allocating subjects?

There are four major ways to randomly allocate subjects:

1 Randomization with equal allocation.
2 Blocked randomization.

[4] Connors, A. F., Speroff, T., Dawson, N. V., *et al.* "The effectiveness of right-heart catheterization in the initial care of critically ill patients." *JAMA* **276** (1996): 889–97.
[5] Sandham, J. D., Hull, R. D., Brant, R. F., *et al.* "A randomized, controlled trial of the use of pulmonary artery catheters in high-risk surgical patients." *N. Engl. J. Med.* **348** (2003): 5–14.
[6] Coats, A. J. "Clinical trials, treatment guidelines and real life". *Int. J. Cardiol.* **73** (2000): 205–7.

3 Stratified randomization.
4 Randomization with unequal allocation.

Most studies are performed with equal allocation (simple randomization), i.e., an equal number of subjects are randomized to each group. Equal allocation is simple and provides maximum power. Although randomization with equal allocation will result in approximately equal numbers of subjects in each group, you could get by chance more subjects in one group than another. This can be an issue with small studies (< 20 subjects per group) and can be avoided with blocked randomization.

With blocked randomization, subjects are randomized in small blocks (e.g., four or six subjects), thereby guaranteeing an equal number of subjects in each group. With two groups (for example, A and B) randomization in blocks of four could result in the following patterns: AABB, ABAB, BABA, ABBA, BAAB, BBAA. In all of these patterns, if you randomize four subjects, you would have two subjects in group A and two subjects in group B. In contrast, with randomization of four subjects without blocking you could have a pattern of AAAA or BBBB.

As with unblocked randomization, blocked randomization does not guarantee that important prognostic factors will be balanced. Blocked randomization only makes sense in small studies when an imbalance in the number of subjects per group would decrease power. For example, if you were randomizing 24 patients, you would not want to risk having 10 in one group and 14 in another.

Both equal allocation and blocked randomization may result in imbalances in the prognostic characteristics across study groups (Section 4.2). This problem can be avoided with stratified randomization.

As implied by the name, stratified randomization means randomizing subjects within certain strata so as to be certain to balance groups across important prognostic factors. For example, if it were important to have an equal number of men and women in your study because gender has a strong influence on the outcome or the effectiveness of the intervention, you could stratify your randomization by gender.

Although stratification may sound sensible, it requires knowledge of the important baseline characteristics prior to the study, is unworkable for more than a few baseline characteristics, and requires you to incorporate the stratification in your analysis, thus complicating data analysis. In practice stratified randomization is used only in (1) small studies with strong prognostic factors, (2) trials where there will be interim analyses (Section 9.4) with small numbers of patients, or (3) equivalence and non-inferiority studies (Section 9.2).[7]

[7] Kernan, W. N., Viscoli, C. M., Makuch, R. W., Brass, L. M., and Horwitz, R. I. "Stratified randomization for clinical trials." *J. Clin. Epidemiol.*, **52** (1999): 19–26.

Randomization with unequal allocation is essentially a simple randomization except that instead of randomizing patients one-to-one to the different groups, you randomize them in an unequal fashion such as two-to-one favoring one group. Generally, unequal randomization is chosen so that a higher proportion of subjects receive the treatment (in a treatment versus placebo study) or a new treatment (in a new treatment versus conventional treatment study).

> Unequal allocation decreases power and may undermine equipoise.

The advantage of unequal randomization is that it might provide greater incentive for some subjects to enter a treatment trial if they feel that they have a better than equal chance of receiving the treatment (say 66%). Also, by having more subjects in the treatment arm you will learn more about side effects associated with a novel treatment. The problem with unequal randomization is that it decreases the power of your study. Also, unequal randomization suggests that the investigator believes that one arm is superior to the other arms. This is inconsistent with the principle of equipoise.

> Unless you have a strong reason to do otherwise, perform a simple randomization with equal allocation.

Overall, unless you have a strong reason to do otherwise, perform a simple randomization with equal allocation.

4.5 What is clustered (group) randomization?

> Cluster randomization means that groups, rather than individuals, are randomized.

It is possible to conduct a randomized study by randomizing groups of participants, rather than individuals. This type of randomization is referred to as group or cluster randomization.

Commonly randomized groups include schools, medical practices, clinics, hospitals, businesses, and communities. (Table 4.1).

> It is often easier to randomize groups than individuals.

Cluster randomization has several advantages over randomization of individuals.[8] Often, it is easier to randomize groups than individuals. For example, to test an intervention to promote healthful eating and exercise among school-age children, consider how much easier it would be to randomize 20 schools to either an educational intervention or to no intervention than to individually randomize the students within the school. Remember that to randomize the students you would need to obtain their informed consent prior to their randomization. If you randomize the schools, you can obtain informed consent from the students and their families after randomization. Knowing which arm of the study they are in may increase participation.

Continuing with the same example, consider how much easier it would be to implement an intervention in 10 schools than to create an intervention in

---

[8] Donner, A. and Klar, N. "Pitfalls of and controversies in cluster randomization trials." *Am. J. Public Health* **94** (2004): 416–22.

Table 4.1. Examples of clustered randomization.

Types of clusters that can be randomized	Example
Schools	Eighteen schools were randomized to one of three groups: classroom-based intervention to improve cardiac health for all 3rd and 4th graders, a risk-based intervention only for students with cardiovascular risk factors, or no intervention.[a]
Medical practices or clinics or hospitals or nursing homes	Thirty-one hospitals were randomized either to an intervention designed to increase breastfeeding or to usual practice.[b]
Businesses	Thirty-six pharmacies were randomized to one of three study groups: pharmaceutical care, peak flow monitoring only, or usual care for patients with asthma.[c]
Communities	Twelve rural communities were randomized either to a community intervention to reduce inappropriate antibiotic use plus clinical support systems for clinicians in that area or to just the community intervention.[d]

[a] Harrell, J. S., McMurray, R. G., Gansky, S. A., *et al.* "A public health vs a risk-based intervention to improve cardiovascular health in elementary school children: The cardiovascular health in children study." *Am. J. Public Health* **89** (1999): 1529–35.

[b] Kramer, M. S., Chalmers, B., Hodnett, E. D., *et al.* "Promotion of breastfeeding intervention trial (PROBIT): a randomized trial in the Republic of Belarus." *JAMA* **285** (2001): 413–20.

[c] Weinberger, M., Murray, M. D., Marrero, D. G., *et al.* "Effectiveness of pharmacist care for patients with reactive airways disease: a randomized controlled trial." *JAMA* **288** (2002): 1594–602.

[d] Samore, M. H., Bateman, K., Alder, S. C., *et al.* "Clinical decision support and appropriateness of antimicrobial prescribing." *JAMA* **294** (2005): 2305–14.

all 20 schools and have only the randomized half of the students be exposed to the intervention.

Besides being easier to perform, clustered randomization makes it less likely that the control group will be exposed to (contaminated by) the intervention. Using the school example, if you randomized students within schools imagine how hard it would be to keep the children randomized to a control group from hearing the messages of the intervention from their fellow schoolmates.

Perhaps the best reason to do a clustered randomization is because the intervention is operating on a group (not individual) level. For example, to perform an intervention to improve hospital or clinic performance, it wouldn't make sense to randomize individual patients or doctors because the intervention is aimed at improving care within the entire hospital or clinic.

> Conducting an intervention may be easier with cluster randomization than randomization of individuals.

> Cluster randomization is less likely to result in contamination of the groups.

For example, Shafer and colleagues sought to increase the screening rate for chlamydia among sexually active adolescent girls.[9] Five clinics were randomized to perform the intervention and five were randomized to provide usual care. In the intervention clinics, administrators, medical assistants, nurses, and practitioners were engaged in redesigning clinic flow to increase screening rates; the group decided that the best way to increase screening would be to ask all adolescents to leave a urine specimen at registration, and let the practitioners decide later which ones to send. The investigators found that the screening rate for sexually active adolescent girls was higher in the intervention clinics than in the usual care clinics.

Remember that whether you are randomizing groups or individuals, to achieve an equal balance of baseline characteristics there must be a sufficient number of units to randomize. If, for example, you randomize only two cities, your sample is too small for randomization to balance baseline characteristics. To illustrate: consider randomizing one of two cities to an intervention or a control group. The two cities that have agreed to participate and accept randomization are: New York City and New Delhi. No matter which city is randomized to the intervention, the two cities and the participants within them will be different. Conversely, if you randomize two similar cities, the cities and the participants in them will be similar on measured characteristics but not because of the randomization.

> For clustered randomization to work there must be a sufficient number of clusters.

Data from a clustered randomized study, or any clustered study (nonrandomized clustered studies are discussed in Section 5.4.B), must be analyzed differently than data from a nonclustered study. Specifically, the correlation between clustered individuals must be incorporated into the analysis.[10]

4.6 What can be randomized besides individuals or clusters of individuals?

Because of the unique ability of randomization to produce groups that are comparable with respect to both measured and unmeasured characteristics, investigators who cannot randomize individuals or clusters of individuals will sometimes identify some other feature to randomize. For example, O'Donnell and colleagues were interested in determining the impact of video-based education on patients seen at an STD clinic.[11] They compared three treatment

---

[9] Shafer, M. B., Tebb, K. P., Pantell, R. H., *et al.* "Effect of a clinical practice improvement intervention on chlamydial screening among adolescent girls." *JAMA* **288** (2002): 2846–52.

[10] Two commonly used techniques for analyzing clustered data are generalized estimating equations and mixed-effects models. For more on these techniques see: Chapter 6, footnote 22.

[11] O'Donnell, L. N., Doval, A. S., Duran, R., and O'Donnell, C. "Video-based sexually transmitted disease patient education: its impact on condom acquisition." *Am. J. Public Health* **85** (1995): 817–22.

conditions: video education, video education plus group discussion, and control. Because it was logistically difficult to randomize patients within a clinic setting, treatment conditions were assigned on random days of clinic operation. In other words, on any given day subjects were enrolled into only one condition and that condition was chosen randomly. Although the investigators could have prevented bias by randomizing STD clinics (clustered randomization), that would have required a much more complicated study with multiple sites and investigators. Randomizing days was an economical and practical solution.

One criticism of this type of design is that study staff would know prior to the enrollment of any individual what treatment assignment they would get. This is not true when you randomize individuals.

Another feature that may be randomized is duplicative body parts. For example, Kiel and colleagues randomly assigned nursing home residents to wear a one-sided hip protector on the left hip or the right hip.[12] The randomization of hip was done at the level of the nursing home (clustered randomization) to make it easier for the staff to remember which side of the body to place the pad. Unfortunately, the incidence rate of hip fracture was similar for the protected and unprotected hips.

4.7 When should subjects and researchers be masked (blinded) to treatment assignment?

> Mask (blind) subjects and investigators to treatment assignment whenever possible.

Whenever possible!

As we have discussed, randomization prevents bias in the treatment assignment (Section 4.2). However, if the subjects or the researchers know the assignment (open label) bias enters! Why? Because subjects and researchers will have expectations – whether true or not – about the different treatments being studied.

For example, in an active drug trial, the person who knows they have received the active drug may feel better immediately – even before taking the first dose – just knowing that they will be getting the active drug. The person randomized to the higher-dose arm of a low-dose/high-dose trial may experience side effects because they know that they are receiving a high dose of the medication.

Investigators may be equally influenced. Those who believe that a particular intervention is efficacious may unconsciously perceive those who are

---

[12] Kiel, D. P., Magaziner, J., Zimmerman, S., *et al.* "Efficacy of a hip protector to prevent hip fracture: the HIP PRO randomized controlled trial." *JAMA* **298** (2007): 413–22.

randomized to that intervention to be doing better. This can cause measurement error, especially if the measurements can be affected by how a question is worded, or how an answer is interpreted, or the perception of the observers.

These problems can be avoided by masking subjects and researchers to treatment assignment. This is called a double-masked (blinded) study.

Given the advantages of masking, why not mask subjects in all trials? The answer is that in many trials it is impossible. For example, it is not possible to mask subjects to whether they receive a behavioral counseling session or a housing voucher or a telephone follow-up. Some interventions, such as surgery, can theoretically be blinded, but raise difficult ethical issues.[13] In other cases, subjects may only be willing to participate if the study is open label.

If you can't mask treatment assignment, consider what strategies you can employ to decrease bias due to subjects or investigators knowing the treatment assignment. For subjects, it is important to emphasize to them that it is not known which treatment is better and that's why it is being studied.

To decrease bias from knowledge of treatment by researchers use objective markers, whenever possible. For example, use an automatic blood pressure monitor to measure blood pressure. Any materials that can be assessed without the subjects' presence (e.g., X-ray) should be read by practitioners who do not know the treatment assignment or even the hypothesis of the study.

> Double-masked (blind) means neither the subject nor the investigator knows what treatment the subject is receiving.

> When possible, have materials evaluated by practitioners who do not know treatment assignment or the study hypothesis.

4.8 How do I account for subjects who do not adhere to their treatment?

In a randomized clinical trial there will invariably be subjects who are assigned to a treatment but never take a dose, or who stop taking the treatment because of side effects or because they don't like it, or who are assigned to the placebo group but on their own initiative cross over and take the active treatment. (If you are thinking this can't happen if subjects are blinded to treatment assignment: think again. Subjects are known to send their study medications for drug testing and then start the active treatment if they find out they were randomized to placebo.)

The problems of stopping or switching treatment are not unique to randomized trials. In fact, it is even more common in nonrandomized observational trials because in everyday life patients often stop taking their medicines or switch to a new one. We expect this in observational trials. But the consequences are greater in randomized controlled trials because those who stop taking their randomized treatment, or cross over into one of the study arms, undermine the advantages of randomization.

---

[13] Horng, S. and Miller, F. G. "Is placebo surgery unethical?" *N. Engl. J. Med.* **347** (2002): 137–9.

Subjects who do not adhere to their randomized treatment undermine the advantages of randomization.

Remember that the reason we randomize subjects is to eliminate bias; this enables us to ascribe differences that occur between the groups during the study to the intervention. However, the factors that lead to not complying with treatment, or crossing over to the other treatment arm, are anything but random. Therefore, if you exclude persons who do not take their assigned treatment or reclassify such persons based on their actual behavior you are introducing bias into the randomized groups.

Excluding or reclassifying persons who do not take their randomized treatment introduces bias into the trial.

Rather than excluding or reclassifying subjects who do not adhere to their treatment, analyze your data as if the subject received their assigned treatment (or placebo) to the end of the study. This is called an intention-to-treat analysis.[14]

Intention-to-treat analysis is necessary to maintain the advantages of randomization. In addition intention-to-treat analysis protects against treatments appearing more favorable than they are. Why? Because dropouts and cross-overs occur for a reason – typically because subjects are not happy with how things are going. Therefore we would expect that people who drop out would not do as well as subjects who stay in the study.

Intention-to-treat means analyzing the data such that subjects are counted as members of their originally assigned group, no matter what happens during the study period.

Besides maintaining the randomization, the results of an intention-to-treat analysis are more informative to clinicians starting patients on a regimen because at the outset we do not know whether a patient will comply or not.

Intention-to-treat analysis maintains the advantages of randomization.

That being said, it is sometimes important to see the results from those subjects who actually adhered to the study. This is called a per-protocol analysis. Per-protocol analyses typically exclude persons who were never exposed to the intervention or were insufficiently exposed (e.g., took less than 85% of the drug in a medication trial). This has the advantage that if people were not sufficiently exposed to the intervention to benefit, including them in the intervention arm dilutes the overall impact of the intervention.

Per-protocol analyses include only those persons who followed the protocol.

One type of per-protocol analysis is an as-treated analysis. An as-treated analysis groups subjects based on the treatment they received, rather than the group to which they were randomized. As you can imagine, if you have a large number of subjects who cross over into the other arm, an intention-to-treat analysis will not well characterize the benefits and the risks of the different arms (because the groups as randomized are a mixture of the arms).

An as-treated analysis compares subjects based on the treatment they actually took.

This potential role of an as-treated analysis is well illustrated by a trial of surgical versus non-operative treatment of lumbar disk herniation.[15] In this clinical trial, subjects were randomized to surgery or to non-operative care

---

[14] Ellenberg, J. H. "Intent-to-treat analysis versus as-treated analysis." *Drug Info. J.* **30** (1996): 535–44. Available at www.diahome.org/content/abstract/1996/dj302616.pdf.

[15] Weinstein, J. N., Tostson, T. D., Lurie, J. D., *et al.* "Surgical vs nonoperative treatment for lumbar disk herniation." *JAMA* **296** (2006): 2441–50.

Table 4.2. Comparisons of subjects who received their assigned treatment to those who did not, for both those assigned to surgery and those assigned to non-operative treatment.

	Assigned to surgery No. (%)			Assigned to non-operative treatment No. (%)		
	Surgery (*n* = 140)	No surgery (*n* = 92)	*P* value	Surgery (*n* = 107)	No surgery (*n* = 133)	*P* value
Age, mean, y	40	44	0.01	42	44	0.21
Annual income <$50 000, %	47	29	0.01	56	41	0.02
Pain with straight leg raise (ipsilateral), %	67	53	0.05	67	56	0.11
Herniation level,%						
L2–3/L3–4	3	13	0.01	5	8	0.45
L4–5	36	33		38	33	
L5–S1	61	54		57	58	
Bodily pain, mean*	24	32	0.002	24	29	0.03
Physical function, mean*	36	46	0.003	33	44	<0.001
Disability index, mean**	52	41	<0.001	52	42	<0.001
Sciatica indices, mean						
Frequency	16	15	0.14	17	15	0.009
Bothersomeness	16	15	0.10	16	14	0.001
Satisfaction with symptoms: very dissatisfied, %	89	64	<0.001	86	70	0.005
Self-assessed health trend: getting worse, %	41	26	0.02	41	26	0.02

* Higher score is better.
** Lower score is better.
Data from Weinstein, J. N., *et al.* "Surgical vs nonoperative treatment for lumbar disk herniation." *JAMA* **296** (2006): 2441–50.

(e.g., physical therapy, nonsteroidal anti-inflammatory medications). At two years only 140 (57%) of the 245 subjects randomized to surgery actually had surgery; meanwhile 107 (42%) of the 256 randomized to non-operative care had crossed over and had surgery!

As you can see in Table 4.2, the crossovers were not random. Among those assigned to surgery, those who actually had the surgery were significantly younger, of lower income, more likely to have pain with straight leg raise, more likely to have disk herniation at a lower level, in greater pain, in worse physical function, in greater disability, more dissatisfied with their symptoms, and more likely to assess themselves as getting worse. There were also many statistically significant differences within the non-operative treatment group between those who did and did not have surgery.

Although having so many subjects crossing over to the other treatment arm may seem extreme, this is the real world of randomized trials comparing surgical treatments to medical treatments (i.e., it is natural that people might decide – even

Table 4.3. Comparison of outcomes in patients randomized to surgery to those randomized to non-operative care, intention-to-treat analysis.

	Surgery ($n = 186$)	Non-operative ($n = 187$)	Treatment effect (95% CI)
Bodily pain, mean*	40.3	37.1	3.2 (–2.0 to 8.4)
Physical function, mean*	35.9	35.9	0 (–5.4 to 5.5)
Disability index, mean**	–31.4	–28.7	–2.7 (–7.4 to 1.9)

* Higher score is better.
** Lower score is better.
Data from Weinstein, J. N., *et al.* "Surgical vs nonoperative treatment for lumbar disk herniation." *JAMA* **296** (2006): 2441–50.

Table 4.4. Comparison of intent-to-treat and as-treated analysis.

	Intention-to-treat (surgery vs. non-operative care) treatment effect (95% CI)	As-treated (surgery vs. non-operative care) treatment effect (95% CI)
Bodily pain, mean*	3.2 (–2.0 to 8.4)	15.0 (10.9 to 19.2)
Physical function, mean*	0 (–5.4 to 5.5)	17.5 (13.6 to 21.5)
Disability index, mean**	–2.7 (–7.4 to 1.9)	–15.0 (–18.3 to –11.7)

* Higher score is better.
** Lower score is better.
Data from Weinstein, J. N., *et al.* "Surgical vs nonoperative treatment for lumbar disk herniation." *JAMA* **296** (2006): 2441–50.

if they were unsure what would be best at the start of a trial – that they really did or did not want surgery; or their condition may have changed after randomization in a way that made them strongly favor one treatment over the other).

Nonetheless, the authors were true to the principle that the primary analysis should be intention-to-treat. As you can see in Table 4.3, using an intention-to-treat analysis, those subjects initially assigned to surgery had less pain and less disability. Unfortunately, although two of the three primary outcomes favored the surgery group (the third physical function showed no change) the confidence intervals all included zero, consistent with no difference between the groups.

You may be wondering, since this is an intention-to-treat analysis, why the sample size for the surgery group is 186 instead of 245 and the sample size for the non-operative care is 187 instead of 256. Good question! Remember that intention-to-treat analysis cannot incorporate subjects who were not evaluated for the outcome in question because they withdrew, were lost to follow-up or died (for this you need to censor observations; see Section 6.4.G).

Although it was not the primary analysis, the authors reported the as-treated analysis results. As you can see in Table 4.4 the as-treated analysis shows a much stronger benefit for surgery than the intention-to-treat. In fact, in the as-treated analysis the differences between the surgery and the non-operative group are statistically significant. This is consistent with the possibility that surgery is more effective than non-operative care but the effect is diluted by all the people in the surgical group who did not have surgery and all the people in the non-operative group who had surgery. Nonetheless, the study cannot be considered to conclusively favor surgery.

Nonrandomized studies

5.1 What are nonrandomized studies?

Nonrandomized intervention studies refer to a diverse group of studies that evaluate interventions without randomizing subjects to receive or not receive the intervention. They are often referred to as quasi-experimental studies (quasi- meaning resembling). I prefer the term nonrandomized intervention study because it allows inclusion of studies that do not resemble experiments.

Unlike randomized trials, which must be planned prospectively, nonrandomized studies may be planned, or they may be designed after the intervention has occurred. Nonrandomized studies may or may not have a control group.

5.2 Why perform nonrandomized studies?

Several common scenarios in which nonrandomized designs should be performed along with examples are shown in Table 5.1.

What the first four scenarios in Table 5.1 have in common is that they are circumstances in which randomization is not ethical or practical.

> Perform nonrandomized studies when randomization is unethical or impractical.

For example, Raschke and colleagues developed a computerized system to alert physicians when a patient of theirs was prescribed a medication that could result in an adverse drug event (e.g., a patient receiving digoxin with a low serum potassium level).[1] Theoretically, the investigators could have randomized the doctors to receive or not receive the alerts, or have randomized patients to have their doctors receive alerts or not, or have randomized events (e.g., each time the computer recognized a potential drug event it could be programmed to send or not send a warning on a random basis). However, the investigators felt it would be unethical to not send a warning to physicians each time the computer identified a potential adverse event.

Instead, the investigators evaluated the effect of their system by assessing whether clinicians took action after receiving an alert. Although the study did

---

[1] Raschke, R. A., Gollihare, B., Wunderlich, T. A., *et al.* "A computer alert system to prevent injury from adverse drug events." *JAMA* **280** (1998): 1317–20.

Table 5.1. Common scenarios for performing nonrandomized studies.

Scenario	Example
Comparison of patients before and after an intervention in settings where it is unethical, difficult, or unnecessary to obtain a control group.	Impact of a computer alert system for detecting adverse drug events.[a]
Comparison of patients receiving an intervention to those who receive a different intervention or no intervention, when it is unethical or unfeasible to randomize patients.	Effect of a community mobilization to decrease cardiovascular risk factors.[b]
Changes occurring after passage of a law or creation of a new program.	Association of an indoor smoking ban with incidence of acute coronary syndrome.[c]
Detection of a side effect that is rare or occurs long after the intervention.	Relationship of use of antipsychotic medicines with sudden death in a study linking prescription records to death certificates.[d]
Generalization of a finding that has been established in a randomized trial.	Warfarin is as effective for non-valvular atrial fibrillation when used in clinical settings as in randomized clinic settings.[e]

[a] Raschke, R. A., Gollihare, B., Wunderlich, T. A., *et al.* "A computer alert system to prevent injury from adverse drug events." *JAMA* **280** (1998): 1317–20.

[b] Carleton, R. A., Lasater, T. M., Assaf, A. R., *et al.* "The Pawtucket Heart Health Program: community changes in cardiovascular risk factors and projected disease risk." *Am. J. Public Health* **85** (1995): 777–85.

[c] Pell, J. P., Haw, S., Cobbe, S., *et al.* "Smoke-free legislation and hospitalizations for acute coronary syndrome." *N. Engl. J. Med.* **359** (2008): 482–91.

[d] Ray, W. A., Meredith, S., Thapa, P. B., Meador, K. G., Hall, K., and Murray, K. T. "Antipsychotics and the risk of sudden cardiac death." *Arch. Gen. Psychiatry* **58** (2001): 1161–7.

[e] Go, A. S., Hylek, E. M., Chang, Y., *et al.* "Anticoagulation therapy for stroke prevention in atrial fibrillation: how well do randomized trials translate into clinical practice?" *JAMA* **290** (2003): 2685–92.

not have a control group this was not a major limitation because it is reasonable to assume that if physicians made changes based on the alerts, the alerts were helpful.

In other situations, it is critical to have a control group even if the control group is not randomized because of the possibility that changes seen in the intervention group are due to factors other than the intervention. For example, Carleton and colleagues conducted a community education study to decrease cardiovascular disease.[2] The intervention involved mobilizing the community

[2] Carleton, R. A., Lasater, T. M., Assaf, A. R., *et al.* "The Pawtucket Heart Health Program: community changes in cardiovascular risk factors and projected disease risk." *Am. J. Public Health* **85** (1995): 777–85.

of Pawtucket, Rhode Island, including individuals, community organizations, public and private schools, large work sites, supermarkets, restaurants, and city government, in a variety of educational programs.

Community mobilizations can only be randomized if you have the resources to perform the mobilization in a large enough number of communities (and observe an equally large number of communities where the intervention is not being performed) such that your sample size of communities (not individuals) will be large enough to produce comparable groups. This is rarely feasible and most community mobilizations do not randomize communities but instead choose comparison communities. In the case of the Pawtucket study they used a single comparison city. They found that following the intervention there were decreases in cholesterol, blood pressure, and smoking prevalence in Pawtucket residents, but similar decreases occurred in the comparison community. In this case, having a control group was critical in demonstrating that the changes were not due to the intervention.

Laws usually can be evaluated only with a nonrandomized design.

A common situation for performing a nonrandomized study is evaluation of a new law or government program. In these cases, randomization is rarely an option. Instead, investigators often look for an area of the country that has not passed a similar law or developed a similar program. For example, in 2006 all indoor smoking in public places was banned in Scotland. Pell and colleagues evaluated the impact of the legislation by assessing trends in hospitalizations for acute coronary syndrome.[3] In the period following passage of the legislation, hospital admissions for acute coronary syndrome decreased by 17% compared to the period before the legislation. To assess the likelihood that this drop was due to factors other than the smoking ban, the investigators performed a similar review of hospitalizations in England. No similar ban was in place in England at that time and the decrease in acute coronary syndrome was only 4%.

Nonrandomized studies may be necessary to detect side effects that are rare or occur long after treatment (long latency). In such cases randomized studies may not be feasible because of the number of people who would have to be enrolled or because of the length of time that the trial would have to run. For example, sudden death in association with the use of antipsychotics has been reported. However, sudden death occurs in the absence of antipsychotic drug use, raising the question of whether the rate of sudden death is higher among persons taking antipsychotics than among those not on these medications. If one were to try to answer this question with a randomized controlled trial,

---

[3] Pell, J. P., Haw, S., Cobbe, S., *et al.* "Smoke-free legislation and hospitalizations for acute coronary syndrome." *N. Engl. J. Med.* **359** (2008): 482–91.

Table 5.2. Association between use of antipsychotics and sudden death.

Characteristic	Current use			
	Moderate dose	Low dose	Past year only	Non-user
Person-years of follow-up	26 749	31 864	37 881	1 186 501
Sudden cardiac deaths	46	51	53	1 337
Rate per 10 000 person-years	26.9	14.4	15.7	11.3
Adjusted rate ratio	2.39	1.30	1.20	1
95% confidence interval	1.77–3.22	0.98–1.72	0.91–1.58	(reference)

Data from: Ray, W. A., *et al.* "Antipsychotics and the risk of sudden cardiac death." *Arch. Gen. Psychiatry* **58** (2001): 1161–7.

tens of thousands of patients would need to be enrolled because sudden death is rare.

Instead Ray and colleagues answered the question using a nonrandomized design.[4] The investigators linked Medicaid files (which included prescription records) to death certificates to compare the frequency of sudden death among persons taking moderate-dose antipsychotics, persons taking low-dose antipsychotics, those who previously took antipsychotics, and non-users of antipsychotics.

Note in the first line of Table 5.2 the large number of person-years in each of the categories. This is a major asset for the study because of the small number of events (line 2) and the low rate of events per 10 000 person-years (line 3). With a small sample size differences between the groups would be hard to detect. In fact, prior randomized studies comparing antipsychotics to placebo had too few patients to identify this rare side effect. With this large observational sample the investigators demonstrated that sudden death was significantly higher among moderate users of antipsychotics than among non-users of antipsychotics.

> Nonrandomized studies are valuable for replicating the findings of a randomized controlled trial in a real-world setting.

The fifth indication for performing a nonrandomized study is to increase generalization of a finding. Sometimes an intervention has been proven to work in a randomized clinical trial (efficacy trial), but there are concerns as to whether it would work in a real-world setting (effectiveness trial) (Section 2.2.C). This is especially true of interventions that are complicated or require a lot of cooperation on the part of subjects.

For example, several randomized controlled trials have demonstrated that persons with atrial fibrillation and nonvalvular heart disease should receive anticoagulation with warfarin to prevent ischemic strokes. Although the prevalence of bleeding is higher in persons taking warfarin the extra risk has

[4] Ray, W. A., Meredith, S., Thapa, P. B., Meador, K. G., Hall, K., and Murray, K. T. "Antipsychotics and the risk of sudden cardiac death." *Arch. Gen. Psychiatry* **58** (2001): 1161–7.

been shown to be worth the benefit in these tightly controlled research studies. However, in clinical practice warfarin is a difficult drug to manage. It has a narrow therapeutic window: incorrectly taking an extra dose or missing a dose, or changes in diet, can result in wide swings in the level of anticoagulation. Also, few elderly persons were included in the clinical trials, despite the fact that atrial fibrillation is common in the elderly and it is elders in whom bleeds can be particularly a problem due to the higher incidence of falls.

To determine whether the benefits and side effects of warfarin in clinical practice were similar to those seen in research settings, Go and colleagues reviewed medical, pharmaceutical, and laboratory records of 11 526 patients with non-valvular atrial fibrillation and no contraindication to anticoagulation who were enrolled in a staff-model health maintenance organization (Kaiser Permanente).[5] They found that the benefits of warfarin in preventing ischemic stroke, as well as the increased risk of intracranial hemorrhage, were similar in magnitude to those seen in randomized studies. This gives a strong rationale for anticoagulating patients with nonvalvular atrial fibrillation who have no contraindication to it.

5.3 What are the disadvantages of nonrandomization?

> With nonrandomized designs groups may differ at baseline.

The major disadvantage of nonrandomized designs is that the groups may differ at baseline in ways that will confound your results. Confounding occurs in an intervention study when a factor is associated with whether or not the participant receives the intervention and is causally related to outcome (Figure 5.1).

To illustrate the impact of confounding in a nonrandomized study let's look at a study assessing the efficacy of influenza vaccination for elderly persons living in the community.[6] Using administrative databases of persons enrolled in a health maintenance organization, the researchers identified persons who had received vaccination and compared them to those who had not. As you can see in Table 5.3, the mean number of hospitalizations due to respiratory infections during two influenza seasons is higher in the vaccination group. From these data we would conclude that the vaccine is not effective in decreasing hospitalizations, and may actually increase hospitalizations due to respiratory infections.

However, as is usually the case in nonrandomized studies, the two groups differed on a number of baseline characteristics, including frequency of coronary heart disease, chronic lung disease, diabetes, vasculitis or rheumatologic

---

[5] Go, A. S., Hylek, E. M., Chang, Y., *et al.* "Anticoagulation therapy for stroke prevention in atrial fibrillation: how well do randomized trials translate into clinical practice?" *JAMA* **290** (2003): 2685–92.

[6] Nichol, K. L., Margolis, K. L., Wuorenma, J., and Sternberg, T. V. "The efficacy and cost effectiveness of vaccination against influenza among elderly persons living in the community." *N. Engl. J. Med.* **331** (1994): 778–84.

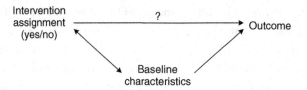

Figure 5.1   Confounding in an intervention study.

Table 5.3. Hospitalizations per 1000 elderly persons for acute and chronic respiratory conditions among vaccine recipients and non-recipients during two seasons of influenza.

	1991–1992 Vaccination		1992–1993 Vaccination	
	Yes	No	Yes	No
	($n = 15\,288$)	($n = 11\,081$)	($n = 14\,647$)	($n = 11\,979$)
Mean no. of hospitalizations per 1000 persons for acute and chronic respiratory conditions.	31.8	31.0	30.7	26.5

Data from Nichol, K. L., *et al.* "The efficacy and cost effectiveness of vaccination against influenza among elderly persons living in the community." *N. Engl. J. Med.* **331** (1994): 778–84.

> Confounding by indication means that the subject receives the intervention based on factors casually associated with outcome.

disease, and dementia or stroke (Table 5.4). And in most cases the differences favored the no-vaccination group; in other words, the persons receiving the vaccination were sicker. This type of confounding is referred to as confounding by indication. Confounding by indication occurs when a factor is related to the likelihood of a subject receiving an intervention and is causally related to outcome.[7]

In the case of this study, patients who were chronically sicker were more likely to receive influenza vaccine because they and their physicians were more concerned about them becoming seriously ill if they were to develop influenza. (You can also have confounding by contraindication if the treatment is one that is avoided for sicker people, such as surgery.)[8]

---

[7] Confounding by indication should be distinguished from selection bias. Selection bias occurs when a variable influences whether a subject receives an intervention (e.g., region where the subject lives) but is not independently associated with the outcome (generally where you live does not affect your likelihood of disease, unless the disease is due to an environmental exposure). For more on this issue see: Salas, M., Hofman, A., and Stricker B.H. "Confounding by indication: an example of variation in the use of epidemiologic terminology." *Am. J. Epidemiol.* **149** (1999): 981–3.

[8] For more on confounding by indication see: Hak, E., Verheij T. J. M., Grobbee, D. E., Nichol, K. L., and Hoes, A. W. "Confounding by indication in non-experimental evaluation of vaccine effectiveness: the example of prevention of influenza complications." *J. Epidemiol. Community Health* **56**

Table 5.4. Baseline characteristics of patients by vaccination status during two influenza seasons.

	1991–1992 Vaccination			1992–1993 Vaccination		
	Yes	No		Yes	No	
Characteristic	($n = 15\,288$)	($n = 11\,081$)	P value	($n = 14\,647$)	($n = 11\,979$)	P value
Outpatient diagnoses during prior 12 mo. (%)						
Coronary heart disease	15.5	8.9	<0.001	17.1	11.5	<0.001
Chronic lung disease	9.9	5.2	<0.001	10.1	6.4	<0.001
Diabetes	10.8	6.4	<0.001	11.6	7.9	<0.001
Vasculitis or rheumatologic disease	2.0	1.1	<0.001	2.1	1.3	<0.001
Dementia or stroke	2.2	3.9	<0.001	2.4	4.5	<0.001
Inpatient diagnoses during prior 12 mo. (%)						
Coronary heart disease	4.8	2.9	<0.001	5.4	3.7	<0.001
Chronic lung disease	2.6	1.8	<0.001	2.5	2.1	0.06
Pneumonia prior 12 mo. (%)	4.1	2.5	<0.001	4.1	3.4	0.003

Data from: Nichol, K. L., *et al.* "The efficacy and cost effectiveness of vaccination against influenza among elderly persons living in the community." *N. Engl. J. Med.* **331** (1994): 778–84.

Table 5.5. Hospitalizations per 1000 elderly persons for acute and chronic respiratory conditions among vaccine recipients and nonrecipients during two influenza seasons.

	Mean no. of hospitalizations/1000			
	1991–1992 Vaccination		1992–1993 Vaccination	
	Yes	No	Yes	No
Cause of hospitalization	($n = 15\,288$)	($n = 11\,081$)	($n = 14\,647$)	($n = 11\,979$)
Acute and chronic respiratory conditions				
Unadjusted	31.8	31.0	30.7	26.5
Adjusted	23.7	39.0	24.1	33.1
Difference (95% CI)	−15.3 (−22.4 to −8.2)		−9.0 (−16.0 to −2.0)	
P value	<0.001		0.01	

Data from Nichol, K. L., *et al.* "The efficacy and cost effectiveness of vaccination against influenza among elderly persons living in the community." *N. Engl. J. Med.* **331** (1994): 778–84.

As you can see in Table 5.5, when the investigators used multivariable analysis to adjust for baseline differences between the two groups, the rate of hospitalization was significantly higher for those who did not receive the vaccine.

(2002): 951–5. www.jech.bmj.com; Grobbee, D. E. and Hoes, A. W. "Confounding and indication for treatment in evaluation of drug treatment for hypertension." *BMJ* **315** (1997): 1151–4. http://bmj. bmjjournals.com/cgi/content/full/315/7116/1151.

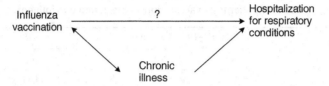

Figure 5.2   Confounding by indication for influenza vaccination.

The 95% confidence intervals for the difference between the hospitalization rates excludes zero. The multivariable analysis tells us a different – and more valid – story about the effectiveness of influenza immunization in preventing hospitalizations due to respiratory disease.

Multivariable analysis is the most commonly used analytic method for dealing with confounding in nonrandomized designs. Stratification – looking for differences within groups – can be used when there are only one or two important differences but this was not the case in this study, where the vaccinated group and the nonvaccinated group differed on a large number of characteristics. And, in fact, it is rare for groups to differ by only one or two factors, and so stratification is not often used to adjust for baseline differences. Other advanced methods of dealing with confounding in nonrandomized studies include propensity analysis, instrumental analysis, and sensitivity analysis (Chapter 7).

There are also ways of achieving comparable baseline groups through the design phase of your study. These are considered in the next section.

5.4 How can I assemble comparable samples in the design phase without randomization?

Two methods for assembling comparable samples in the design phase are matching and identification of similar groups (clusters) of participants.

5.4.A Matching

> Individual matching can be used to create comparable groups.

With individual matching, persons who receive the intervention are matched to persons not receiving the intervention on those variables that are thought to be related to outcome.

For example, Sjostrom and colleagues used an individual matching design to evaluate the effectiveness of bariatric surgery for obesity.[9] Obese subjects were

---

[9] Sjostrom, L., Narbro, K., Sjostrom, C. D., *et al.* "Effects of bariatric surgery on mortality in Swedish obese subjects." *N. Engl. J. Med.* **357** (2007): 741–52; Sjostrom, L., Lindroos, A., Peltonen, M., *et al.*

Table 5.6. Comparison of matched patients self-selecting for surgery or for conventional treatment.

	Surgical treatment ($n = 2010$)	Conventional treatment ($n = 2037$)	P value
Sex (no.)			
Male	590	590	
Female	1420	1447	0.79
Women who were post-menopausal (%)	32	36	0.04
Age at examination (yr)	46	47	<0.001
Daily smoking (%)	28	20	<0.001
Diabetes (%)	7	6	0.12
Weight (kg)	119	117	<0.001
Height (m)	1.7	1.7	0.64
Waist circumference (cm)	124	122	<0.001
Hip circumference (cm)	126	124	<0.001
Systolic blood pressure	141	140	0.25
Triglycerides (mmol/liter)	2.23	2.15	0.09
Cholesterol (mmol/liter)	5.84	5.75	0.004
Current health score	21	23	<0.001
Monotony avoidance score	23	23	0.525
Psychasthenia score	23.9	23.2	<0.001
Quantity of social support	6	6	0.48
Quality of social support	4	4	0.55
Stressful life events	3	2	0.09

Data from: Sjostrom, L., *et al.* "Effects of bariatric surgery on mortality in Swedish obese subjects." *N. Engl. J. Med.* **357** (2007): 741–52.

recruited through the mass media and through primary health care centers, and were asked to complete questionnaires, including stating their preference for surgical treatment or for medical treatment. Subjects who wanted surgery and who were eligible for it were scheduled for the procedure. Those who did not want surgery formed the pool of potential controls.

Using a computer matching algorithm, cases were matched to controls on 18 variables (a case could have more than one match). As you would imagine, if you required that the cases match the controls exactly on 18 variables, such that a case weighing 120.3 kg could only match with a case weighing exactly 120.3 kg, you would have very few matches. Instead, you specify reasonable ranges for each variable; you might, for example, specify that the weight must be within 2 kg. Because the matches are not exact, the groups may still differ significantly from one another on certain variables after matching. This can be seen in Table 5.6.

Groups may still differ after matching.

"Lifestyle, diabetes, and cardiovascular risk factors 10 years after bariatric surgery." *N. Engl. J. Med.* **351** (2004): 2683–93.

After the investigators performed their matching process, the surgery group and the control group were similar on seven variables: sex, prevalence of diabetes, height, systolic blood pressure, monotony avoidance score, quantity of social support, and quality of social support. On the other eleven variables, there remained statistically significant differences, or near significant differences, but many of these differences were not very large. For example, the difference in the average weight between the two groups was only 2.3 kg, and the group choosing the bariatric surgery were heavier, a difference that would be expected to bias against the intervention appearing to be effective.

Nonetheless, because there were significant differences after matching, the investigators used multivariable analysis to adjust for baseline differences between the two matched groups. Adjusting for a number of potential confounders, the investigators found that persons who had bariatric surgery had a lower risk of death (relative hazard 0.73; 95% confidence intervals 0.56–0.95). An important indication of the success of their matching procedure is that the unadjusted risk of death for persons who had undergone bariatric surgery (relative hazard = 0.76; 95% confidence intervals 0.59–0.99) was almost identical to the multivariable result. In other words, although there were significant differences in the two groups after matching, the matching procedure appears to have eliminated confounding, at least for those variables the investigators measured.

> Matched controls should be from the same population.

This study also illustrates another important point about individual matching as a strategy for achieving comparable groups. The cases and controls should be drawn from the same population. In the case of this study, cases and controls were drawn from the population of obese persons responding to the media or being referred by their providers. Drawing cases and controls from different populations (e.g., cases from hospital wards and controls from random-digit dialing) introduces bias.

There are two different strategies for analyzing matched data. If matching is used only to create comparable groups, then standard statistical techniques can be used to analyze the data – this was the case with the study of bariatric surgery. Alternatively, if the individual one-to-one or one-to-x matching is maintained, then the data must be analyzed with methods specific for matched data.[10]

Although matching can be helpful in assembling comparable groups it has disadvantages. There may be cases for which there is no match – requiring the case to be dropped from the sample. Once you match for a variable, you cannot study its impact on the outcome. Finally, if the matched variables are associated

---

[10] Katz, M. H. *Study Design and Statistical Analysis: A Practical Guide for Clinicians.* Cambridge: Cambridge University Press, 2006: pp. 116–9.

with group membership, matching can cause selection bias. For these reasons, most investigators prefer not to match and instead use analytic methods of achieving comparable groups.

5.4.B Identification of comparable clusters (groups)

In Section 4.5, I reviewed clustered (grouped) randomization. However, even without randomization, identifying comparable clusters can be helpful in assembling comparable groups of subjects.

Commonly used clusters for nonrandomized designs with examples are shown in Table 5.7.

You may be wondering why once you have assembled comparable clusters you wouldn't go ahead and randomize them. This would be a superior design from a statistical point of view. There are three reasons for performing a non-randomized cluster study: (1) randomization is too difficult to accomplish or will not be accepted by the target population; (2) your study is taking advantage of a natural experiment and you can't choose the group receiving the intervention; or (3) the number of clusters is too small for randomization to result in comparable groups (Section 4.5).

To illustrate the real-world difficulties of randomizing even within clusters,[11] consider a study designed to assess the effectiveness of vaccination in preventing influenza among children.[12] The investigators identified 11 demographically similar clusters of schools. In the case of seven of the 11 clusters, the intervention school (where the children received the influenza vaccination) was chosen randomly. But in the case of four of the clusters, the school administrators chose which school within the cluster would receive the vaccination. The schools would not allow the use of placebos because they felt that there would be no benefit to the children in receiving placebo. Although a fully randomized, placebo-controlled study would have been a stronger design for proving efficacy of the vaccination, the study would not have happened had the investigators held rigidly to these criteria. As it happened, the study demonstrated that children who received the influenza vaccination were less likely to have a febrile influenza-like illness during the peak influenza week. When the results were limited to those children in schools chosen randomly, vaccination remained effective.

[11] The term "clusters" can be confusing, in part, because there can be different levels of clusters. For example, a school has a cluster of students; a district has a cluster of schools; a state has a cluster of districts, etc. In the case of this study, the choice of which school within the cluster of eligible schools received the intervention was made either randomly or by the administrators.

[12] King, J. C., Stoddard, J. J., Gaglani, M. J., *et al.* "Effectiveness of school-based influenza vaccination." *N. Engl. J. Med.* **355** (2006): 2523–32.

Table 5.7. Nonrandomized designs using clusters.

Potential cluster	Example
Schools	An intervention to improve diet and increase physical activity of students was implemented at six schools; the comparison group was students from eight matched schools.[a]
Towns or cities	An education intervention for adults on cardiovascular disease prevention was implemented in three communities; the comparison group was adults in three communities matched on size and type.[b]
Hospitals or clinics or doctors	An intervention to reduce antibiotic prescribing for acute bronchitis in adults was implemented in one primary care practice; the comparison groups were one clinic that received only a limited intervention, and two clinics that provided usual care.[c]
Businesses	An intervention to improve nutrition of shoppers was implemented in 20 supermarkets; the comparison group was 20 supermarkets matched with regard to neighborhood racial composition, age, occupation, income, proportion of homeowners, and presence of pharmacy in the store.[d]
Neighborhoods, police beats	A multifaceted violence program shows decreased shootings in police beats that received intervention compared to those that did not.[e]

[a] Gortmaker, S. L., Cheung, L. W. Y., Peterson, K. E., *et al.* "Impact of a school-based interdisciplinary intervention on diet and physical activity among urban primary school children." *Arch. Pediatr. Adolesc. Med.* **153** (1999): 975–83.

[b] Luepker, R. V., Murray, D. M., Jacobs, D. R., *et al.* "Community education for cardiovascular disease prevention: risk factor changes in the Minnesota Heart Health Program." *Am. J. Public Health* **84** (1994): 1383–93.

[c] Gonzales, R., Steiner, J. F., Lum, A., and Barrett, P. H. "Decreasing antibiotic use in ambulatory practice: impact of a multidimensional intervention on the treatment of uncomplicated acute bronchitis in adults." *JAMA* **281** (1999): 1512–9.

[d] Rodgers, A. B., Kessler, L. G., Portnoy, B., *et al.* "'Eat for Health': a supermarket intervention for nutrition and cancer risk reduction." *Am. J. Public Health* **84** (1994): 72–6.

[e] *Chicago Project for Violence Prevention.* Fiscal Year 2007 Report to the State of Illinois. August 2007. www.ceasefireillinois.org

As occurs with individual matching, there may be differences between the individuals within matched clusters that require statistical adjustment with multivariable analysis. These methods are discussed in Chapter 7.

Statistical analysis of intervention trials

6.1 How do I test whether my intervention has had a statistically significant effect?

Up until this section, I have not explicitly addressed how to test whether the effect of an intervention is statistically significant. We have, however, covered the basic ingredients.

First, the study hypothesis should be stated in the null. To review, the null hypotheses for the three major questions of intervention studies are:

1 There is no change between the pre-intervention and the post-intervention assessment.
2 The change between the pre-intervention and the post-intervention assessment in the intervention group is no greater than the change in the comparison group.
3 The outcome for the intervention group is no different than that of the comparison group.

Next we use statistics to determine the probability that the null hypothesis is correct. If the probability is very low, we consider the alternative hypothesis: that the intervention is associated with a significant change.

To choose the correct statistic you need to identify:

(a) the nature of your outcome variable,
(b) the number of times you have measured the outcome,
(c) the number of study groups,
(d) whether you need a bivariate test or a multivariable test, and
(e) whether your data are longitudinal cohort or serial cross-sectional.

To help you identify the type of outcome variable you have, I have listed them with examples in Table 6.1.[1]

---

[1] I have not included nominal variables in Table 6.1 because they are infrequently used as outcome variables. For a detailed review of variable types, including how to determine whether an interval variable has a normal distribution see Katz, M. H. *Study Design and Statistical Analysis: A Practical Guide for Clinicians*. Cambridge: Cambridge University Press, 2006: pp. 35–6, 52–9.

Table 6.1. Types of outcome variables.

Type of variable	Description	Example
Interval (continuous), normal distribution	Equal-sized intervals on all parts of the scale are equal. Values on the variable have a bell-shaped distribution.	Blood pressure in a probability sample of the population.
Interval (continuous), non-normal distribution	Equal-sized intervals on all parts of the scale are equal. Values on the variable are not bell-shaped, but may be skewed to the right, to the left, or have a bimodal distribution or a threshold distribution.	Length of hospital stay (typically, the variable will be skewed to the right; the shortest stay is usually less than a day, the mean stay may be 3–4 days, and some patients stay in the hospital for months).
Ordinal	Multiple categories that can be ordered.	NYHA classification of heart failure.
Dichotomous	Two categories.	Alive/dead, heart attack (yes/no).
Time to outcome	Time from start of observation to dichotomous outcome.	Time to death, time to cancer remission.

In terms of number of measurements, the choice of statistic generally depends on whether you have two data points, multiple data points, or a series of data points (e.g., 20 or more); the latter circumstance will be considered in the section on time series (Chapter 8). For choice of statistics, whether you have two study groups or more than two will affect some decisions. Finally, the statistics for longitudinal cohort studies are different than those for cross-sectional studies because with the former the observations are not independent of one another.

To make it easier for you to find the right test, I have organized the statistical sections by these different components: hypothesis 1 is Sections 6.2 and 6.3, hypothesis 2 is Sections 6.4 and 6.5, and hypothesis 3 is Section 6.6. Within each of these sections, I will cover the statistics for the different types of outcome, different numbers of observations, different numbers of groups, and bivariate and multivariable statistics. Because the statistics for longitudinal studies are very different than those for serial cross-sectional studies, I discuss these separately (Sections 6.2 and 6.4 are for longitudinal studies and Sections 6.3 and 6.5 are for serial cross-sectional studies).

6.2 Is the difference between the pre-intervention and the post-intervention assessment statistically significant in a longitudinal study?

The bivariate tests for comparing the difference between the pre-intervention and the post-intervention assessments in longitudinal studies without a control group (one group) are shown in Table 6.2.

I will review the tests for each category of outcome variable in the next four sections.

Table 6.2. Bivariate tests for comparing pre-intervention versus post-intervention assessments in a longitudinal study, no control group.

Outcome measure	Two measurements of outcome over time	Three or more measurements of outcome over time
Interval, normal distribution	Difference between means with 95% confidence intervals. Paired t-test	Repeated measures analysis of variance
Interval, non-normal distribution	Wilcoxon signed-rank test	Friedman test
Ordinal	Wilcoxon signed-rank test	Friedman test
Dichotomous	McNemar's test	Cochran's Q

6.2.A Interval outcome with a normal distribution

When you have a pre-intervention versus post-intervention design, and an interval variable with a normal distribution, the easiest way to demonstrate the difference between the two measurements is to calculate the mean difference (post-intervention mean – pre-intervention mean) and the 95% confidence intervals of that difference. This is an especially satisfying method when the outcome is in clinically meaningful units, such as kilograms of weight, mm of Hg of blood pressure, etc. With variables such as these, the reader quickly gains a sense of whether the difference is clinically meaningful in addition to whether it is statistically significant.

> **TIP**
>
> For outcomes measured in clinically meaningful units, report the mean difference with 95% confidence intervals.

For example, Savoye and colleagues developed a weight management program, Bright Bodies, for overweight children aged 8 to 16 years.[2] The family-based intervention included exercise, nutrition, and behavioral modification. At 6 months, the average weight loss was 2.6 kg (Table 6.3). This gives you a good sense of the average impact of the intervention. The fact that the 95% confidence intervals exclude 1 tells you that the reduction was unlikely to be due to chance. Unfortunately by 12 months the average weight change from baseline was a slight increase. The confidence intervals do not exclude 1, telling you that the change in weight is not statistically significant.

> Paired t-tests are used to compare pre-intervention and post-intervention measurements of normally distributed interval outcomes.

Another way to test whether the difference between a pre- and post-intervention measurement of a normally distributed interval variable is greater than you would expect by chance is to use a paired t-test. For example, Garfinkel and colleagues evaluated whether yoga would relieve the symptoms of carpal tunnel syndrome.[3] They found that there was a significant improvement from

[2] Savoye, M., Shaw, M., Dziura, J., *et al.* "Effects of a weight management program on body composition and metabolic parameters in overweight children: a randomized controlled trial." *JAMA* **297** (2007): 2697–704.

[3] Garfinkel, M. S., Singhal, A., Katz, W. A., *et al.* "Yoga-based intervention for carpal tunnel syndrome: A randomized trial." *JAMA* **280** (1998): 1601–3.

Table 6.3. Weight change among 105 overweight children enrolled in Bright Bodies.

	Baseline	6 months	12 months
Mean weight	87.0 kg	84.4 kg	87.3 kg
Mean change from baseline		−2.6 kg	0.3 kg
95% confidence intervals		−4.2 to −0.9 kg	−1.4 to 2.0 kg

Data from Savoye, M., *et al.* "Effects of a weight management program on body composition and metabolic parameters in overweight children: A randomized controlled trial." *JAMA* **297** (2007): 2697–704.

Table 6.4. Comparison before and after a yoga course (twice a week for 8 weeks).

Variable	n	Mean (SD)		P value
		Pre-course	Post-course	
Grip strength, mmHg	33	161.6 (70.4)	187.4 (68.8)	0.009
Pain, visual analog scale (1–10)	22	5.0 (2.8)	2.9 (2.2)	0.02
Median nerve sensory conduction, ms	35	4.40 (1.5)	3.97 (1.5)	0.18
Median nerve motor conduction, ms	33	4.79 (1.3)	4.27 (1.4)	0.08

Data from Garfinkel, M.S., *et al.* "Yoga-based intervention for carpal tunnel syndrome: A randomized trial." *JAMA* **280** (1998): 1601–3.

pretest to posttest on several measures; specifically, grip strength increased and the amount of pain decreased; there was also a trend toward improvement in the sensory conduction times (faster times are better) (Table 6.4).

The statistical significance of the differences in Table 6.4 are assessed using a paired *t*-test. A paired *t*-test is calculated as the mean change between the paired observations divided by the standard deviation of that change. Large *t* values are associated with small *P* values.

> To compare multiple measurements of a normally distributed interval variable use repeated measures analysis of variance.

When you have more than two measures of a normally distributed interval variable you cannot calculate a mean difference or use a paired *t*-test. Instead use repeated measures analysis of variance.

For example, Taubert and colleagues evaluated the impact of dark chocolate on blood pressure.[4] The changes in blood pressure at 6 weeks, 12 weeks, and 18 weeks from baseline are shown in Table 6.5.

If the *P* value of the repeated measures analysis of variance is statistically significant you can make pairwise comparisons. However, the *P* values from these comparisons must be adjusted for multiple comparisons. The authors of

[4] Taubert, D., Roesen, R., Lehmann, C., Jung, N., and Schomig, E. "Effects of low habitual cocoa intake on blood pressure and bioactive nitric oxide." *JAMA* **298** (2007): 49–60.

Table 6.5. Effect of consumption of dark chocolate on blood pressure.

	Mean change from baseline (mmHg)			P value
	6 weeks	12 weeks	18 weeks	
Systolic	−0.6	−2.4	−2.9	<0.001
Diastolic	−0.3	−1.3	−1.9	<0.001

Data from: Taubert, D., *et al*. "Effects of low habitual cocoa intake on blood pressure and bioactive nitric oxide." *JAMA* **298** (2007): 49–60.

this paper used the Holm method.[5] For example, the decrease in blood pressure between baseline and 6 weeks was not statistically significant ($P = 0.16$) but the decrease between baseline and 12 weeks and the decrease between baseline and 18 weeks were both statistically significant ($P < 0.001$).

The most important aspect of the study is that it provides a handy excuse to eat more chocolate!

6.2.B Non-normally distributed interval variable or ordinal variable

> With a non-normally distributed interval or ordinal outcome, use the Wilcoxon test to compare pre-intervention versus post-intervention scores.

When you have a non-normally distributed interval variable or an ordinal variable and you need to test the difference between the pre-intervention and the post-intervention measurement, use the Wilcoxon signed-rank test.[6] For example, Belfort and colleagues evaluated the effectiveness of the medication pioglitazone for the treatment of steatohepatitis (fatty liver) in diabetics.[7] The investigators found there was significant improvement in all four pathological measures of liver disease following treatment (Table 6.6). Because these measures were ordinal, statistical significance was based on the Wilcoxon signed-rank test.

> Use the Friedman test with a non-normally distributed interval or ordinal outcome at three or more points in time.

When you have a non-normally distributed interval or ordinal outcome at three or more points in time, use the Friedman test. For example, Back and colleagues evaluated the impact of tonsillectomy on erythrocyte sedimentation rate (a measure of inflammation).[8] The medians of the rate are shown in Table 6.7.

The Friedman test was significant at $P < 0.001$, suggesting that the procedure causes an inflammatory host response. As with a repeated measures analysis of

---

[5] Holm, S. "A simple sequentially rejective multiple test procedure." *Scand. J. Stat.* **6** (1979): 65–70.

[6] Wilcoxon signed-rank test is not the same as the Wilcoxon rank sum test, which is also known as the Mann–Whitney test. The Wilcoxon signed-rank test, as with other statistics recommended for using with variables that do not have a normal distribution, is referred to as a non-parametric test.

[7] Belfort, R., Harrison, S. A., Brown, K., *et al*. "A placebo-controlled trial of pioglitazone in subjects with nonalcoholic steatohepatitis." *N. Engl. J. Med.* **355** (2006): 2297–307.

[8] Back, L., Poloheimo, M., Ylikoski, J. "Traditional tonsillectomy compared with bipolar radio-frequency thermal ablation tonsillectomy in adults." *Arch. Otolaryngol. Head Neck Surg.* **127** (2001): 1106–12.

Table 6.6. Histologic findings of liver biopsy specimens before and after treatment with pioglitazone.

	Before treatment n	After treatment n	P value
Steatosis			
0 (<5%)	0	6	<0.001
1 (5–33%)	5	12	
2 (>33–66%)	8	4	
3 (>66%)	13	4	
Ballooning necrosis			
0 (None)	4	13	<0.001
1 (Few balloon cells)	6	7	
2 (Many balloon cells)	16	6	
Lobular inflammation			
0 (0 or 1 focus)	0	6	<0.001
1 (2–4 foci)	5	14	
2 (>4 foci)	21	6	
Fibrosis			
0 (None)	2	5	0.002
1 (Perisinusoidal or periportal)	12	15	
2 (Perisinusoidal and portal/periportal)	5	6	
3 (Bridging fibrosis)	7	0	
4 (Cirrhosis)	0	0	

Data from Belfort, R., *et al.* "A placebo-controlled trial of pioglitazone in subjects with nonalcoholic steatohepatitis." *N. Engl. J. Med.* **355** (2006): 2297–307.

Table 6.7. Median of erythrocyte sedimentation rate following tonsillectomy.

	Pre-operative	Post-operative day 1	Post-operative day 14
Erythrocyte sedimentation rate	4 mm/hr	8 mm/hr	17.5 mm/hr

Data from Back, L., *et al.* "Traditional tonsillectomy compared with bipolar radiofrequency thermal ablation tonsillectomy in adults." *Arch. Otolaryngol. Head Neck Surg.* **127** (2001): 1106–12.

variance, when you have a significant value on the Friedman test, you can make pairwise comparisons by using a method that adjusts for multiple pairwise comparisons. In the case of this study, the investigators used the Dunnet method[9] to show that the change between the pre-operative rate and the rate on the first post-operative day was statistically significant (P <0.05), as was the change between the pre-operative rate and the rate on the 14th post-operative day.

[9] The Dunnet test is used for multiple comparisons when you are comparing different groups to a control. In the case of this study the pre-operative rate serves as the control.

Table 6.8. Health care use at the start of insurance compared to after insurance.

	At the start of insurance %	After insurance %	P value
School-aged children (6–11 years) $n = 58$			
Has provider for checkups	68	93	<0.05
Had a checkup in last year	16	41	<0.05
Had unmet medical need	62	2	<0.05
Adolescents (12–18 years) $n = 63$			
Has provider for checkups	59	93	<0.05
Had a checkup in last year	25	54	<0.05
Had unmet medical need	51	2	<0.05

Data from: Slifkin, R.T., *et al.* "Effect of the North Carolina State Children's Health Insurance Program on beneficiary access to care." *Arch. Pediatr. Adolesc. Med.* **156** (2002): 1223–9.

6.2.C Dichotomous outcome

> McNemar's test is for comparing pre-intervention versus post-intervention scores in the same subjects.

When you have a longitudinal study, a dichotomous outcome, and two data points use McNemar's test to assess whether a significant change has occurred between the pre-intervention and the post-intervention assessments. For example, Slifkin and colleagues evaluated the impact of an insurance program on access to care for children and adolescents.[10] Using McNemar's test the investigators showed that children and adolescents were significantly more likely to have a provider for checkups and to have had a checkup in the last year, and were less likely to have an unmet medical need after the establishment of the insurance program (Table 6.8).

> Cochran's Q is for comparing three or more measures of a dichotomous variable over time.

With three or more measures of a dichotomous outcome over time, use Cochran Q. For example, Fagard and colleagues performed a trial of treatment interruptions for human immunodeficiency virus infection.[11] The theory underlying their study was that increased replication of HIV during treatment interruptions would stimulate the immune response and lead to low viral loads. If this theory were correct then you would expect that over time with an increased number of interruptions, the probability of the viral load being detectable would decrease.

The investigators followed 86 patients who interrupted their treatment at five points in time: weeks 2, 12, 22, 32, and 42. Using a cut-off of viral load > 200 copies, the percent of patients having a detectable viral load was stable,

[10] Slifkin, R. T., Freeman, V. A., and Silberman, P. "Effect of the North Carolina State Children's Health Insurance Program on beneficiary access to care." *Arch. Pediatr. Adolesc. Med.* **156** (2002): 1223–29.

[11] Fagard, C., Oxenius, A., Gunthard, H., *et al.* "A prospective trial of structured treatment interruptions in human immunodeficiency virus infection." *Arch. Intern. Med.* **163** (2003): 1220–6.

ranging from 60% to 66%. The Cochran Q test had a P value of 0.7, indicating no significant change over time in proportion of patients with detectable viral load. Indeed, later studies confirmed that treatment interruptions are not therapeutically beneficial for HIV-infected patients.

6.2.D Multivariable tests for determining whether there is a statistically significant difference between the pre-intervention and the post-intervention assessment in a longitudinal study

> Most analyses of pre-intervention versus post-intervention assessments in a single group do not require multivariable analysis.

In general, most analyses of pre-intervention versus post-intervention assessments in a single group do not require multivariable analysis. Because there is only one group there is no need to adjust for differences between groups: subjects are essentially acting as their own control.

However, at times single-group pre-intervention versus post-intervention studies will use multivariable analysis. The usual reason is to identify additional predictors of the post-intervention assessment besides the fact that the intervention has occurred.

For example, in Section 3.3 I cited a study by Two Feathers and colleagues assessing an intervention to improve diabetes-related outcomes among African-Americans and Latinos.[12] For most of the outcomes of the study there was no control group and the investigators used a pre-intervention versus post-intervention design. Consistent with the above discussion and Table 6.2, pre-intervention changes were evaluated with the Wilcoxon signed-rank test for ordinal variables and interval variables[13] and McNemar's test for dichotomous variables.

To learn more about factors that led to the improved outcomes of their subjects other than the intervention, the investigators conducted two types of multivariable analysis: multiple logistic regression for the two outcomes that were dichotomous (dietary knowledge and following a healthy eating plan) and multiple linear regression for the two outcomes that were linear (number of vegetable servings a day and the glycosylated hemoglobin (Hb_{a1c}) level) (Table 6.9).

The first row shows the relationship between the baseline assessment and the post-intervention assessment for each of the four outcomes. Not surprisingly, the baseline assessments are strongly related to the outcomes. But after adjusting for

[12] Two Feathers, J., Kieffer, E. C., Palmisano, G., *et al.* "Racial and ethnic approaches to community health (Reach) Detroit partnership: Improving diabetes-related outcomes among African American and Latino adults." *Am. J. Public Health.* **95** (2005): 1552–60.

[13] The authors don't state whether their interval variables had a non-normal distribution, but even if they were normally distributed, when you have both ordinal and interval variables it is often easier to use non-parametric statistics with both; there is no harm in using non-parametric statistics with interval variables with a normal distribution, except that non-parametric tests have less power.

Table 6.9. Multivariable analysis of predictors of post-intervention assessment scores for four outcomes.

	Dietary knowledge $n = 107$ OR (95% CI)	Healthy eating plan $n = 106$ OR (95% CI)	Vegetable servings/ day $n = 95$ Regression coefficient	Hb_{alc} $n = 90$ Regression coefficient
Baseline response	4.37 (1.2, 12.8)**	3.48 (1.2, 10.6)*	0.584***	0.691***
Age	0.976 (0.94, 1.01)	0.963 (0.92, 1.01)	0.095	0.059
Gender				
Male	1.1 (0.28, 4.4)	0.96 (0.25, 3.7)	−0.028	0.187*
Female	Referent	Referent		
Race/ethnicity				
African-American	0.16 (0.03, 0.77)*	0.11 (0.02, 0.59)**	−0.099	0.010
Latino	Referent	Referent		
Class 3 attendance	4.2 (1.4, 12.7)**	1.1 (0.19, 6.1)	0.082	...
Dietary knowledge	...	4.2 (1.3, 14.1)*	0.186*	...
Monitoring blood glucose				
0–3 days/wk	...	...	...	Referent
4–7 days/wk	...	...	...	−0.266**
Quality of life	...	...	...	−0.254**

$* P < 0.05$; $** P < 0.01$; $*** P < 0.001$.

Data from: Two Feathers, J., *et al.* "Racial and ethnic approaches to community health (Reach) Detroit partnership: Improving diabetes-related outcomes among African American and Latino adults." *Am. J. Public Health* **95** (2005): 1552–60.

the pre-intervention assessment we can appreciate the other associations with the outcomes. For example, after the intervention African-Americans had significantly less dietary knowledge than Latinos and those who attended the third class had greater dietary knowledge than those who missed the third class. Glycosylated hemoglobin (Hb_{alc}) levels were lower among men, persons who tested their blood glucose frequently, and those with higher quality of life.

6.3 Is the difference between the pre-intervention and the post-intervention assessment statistically significant in a serial cross-sectional study?

With serial cross-sectional studies multivariable analysis is almost always used because of differences between the samples.

The statistical analysis of serial cross-sectional data is both simpler and more complicated than the analysis of longitudinal data. It is simpler because with serial cross-sectional data there is no need to take into account the paired nature of the data as must be done with repeated observations of the same persons. It is more complicated because with serial cross-sectional data multivariable analysis is almost always needed to account for differences in the characteristics of the serial samples.

The statistics for assessing whether differences between pre-intervention and post-intervention assessments are statistically significant in a serial cross-sectional study without a control group are shown in Table 6.10.

Table 6.10. Tests for assessing differences between pre-intervention and post-intervention assessments in a serial cross-sectional study, no control group.

Outcome measure	Two groups bivariate	Three or more groups bivariate	Multivariable analysis
Dichotomous	Chi-squared, Fisher's exact Odds ratio	Chi-squared	Multiple logistic regression
Interval, normal distribution	t-test	ANOVA	Multiple linear regression ANOVA ANCOVA
Interval, non-normal distribution	Mann–Whitney test	Kruskal–Wallis test	–*
Ordinal	Mann–Whitney test	Kruskal–Wallis test	Proportional odds regression

*Attempt to transform the outcome variable so that it fits the assumptions of normality and equal variance.

Jones and colleagues used a serial cross-sectional design to assess whether a community-level intervention was effective at reducing HIV risk behavior in Black men who have sex with men (MSM).[14] The intervention was conducted in three cities; there were no control cities. The intervention consisted of group discussions with opinion leaders and social marketing materials. To assess the impact of the intervention serial samples of Black MSM were drawn prior to the intervention (wave 1) and at three post-intervention points (waves 2–4).

> A significant chi-squared does not tell you where the difference lies.

As you can see in column 1 of Table 6.11, the frequency of unprotected intercourse decreased over the four waves of the study. The chi-square was significant ($P = 0.01$). A significant chi-squared simply tells you that the difference between the expected and observed number of subjects in each cell is unlikely to have occurred by chance. It does *not* tell you where the difference lies. Looking at the four waves it appears that the largest difference is between the first wave and the fourth wave. The chi-squared P value is equal to 0.001 for this comparison.[15]

The odds ratios in the second column basically provide the same information as the first column but in a format that facilitates comparisons with multi-variable models (column 3). The odds ratios in the second column for wave two, three, and four are comparisons to wave one. Note that while the odds ratios for wave two and three are less than one, the confidence intervals cross one and are not significant. The odds ratio for wave four is statistically different from one (the confidence intervals do not cross one), indicating that by wave four the men report that they are significantly less likely to have unprotected intercourse.

Part of why I chose this study to illustrate serial cross-sectional studies is that it demonstrates the strengths and weaknesses of this design. In terms of

---

[14] Jones, K. T., Gray, P., Whiteside, Y. O., *et al.* "Evaluation of an HIV prevention intervention adapted for black men who have sex with men." *Am. J. Public Health* **98** (2008): 1043–50.
[15] For more on chi-squared testing including pairwise comparisons see Katz, M. H. *Study Design and Statistical Analysis: A Practical Guide for Clinicians.* Cambridge: Cambridge University Press, 2006: pp. 77–9.

Table 6.11. Change in frequency in unprotected anal intercourse with male partners over four waves of the study.

	Reported behavior, % (no.)	Unadjusted OR (95% CI)	Adjusted[†] OR (95% CI)
Wave 1	42.1 (119/283)	1.00 (reference)	1.00 (reference)
Wave 2	34.5 (99/287)	0.73 (0.52, 1.02)	0.73* (0.53, 1.00)
Wave 3	36.0 (109/303)	0.77 (0.56, 1.08)	0.77 (0.57, 1.06)
Wave 4	28.7 (77/268)	0.56** (0.39, 0.79)	0.57*** (0.41, 0.80)

[†]OR adjusted for city where survey took place, employment status, and whether the respondent had ever been to jail.
* $P < 0.05$; ** $P < 0.01$; *** $P < 0.001$

strengths, the data in the second column would be much less compelling if it was a pre- versus post-intervention cohort study because of the possibility that subjects were telling the investigators what they wanted to hear (social desirability responses, Section 3.7). Although there are objective markers of unsafe sex (e.g., HIV incidence, STD acquisition) these would have been difficult to incorporate in a study because they occur at low incidence.

In terms of weaknesses, because this is a serial cross-sectional design, subjects interviewed in wave 1 are not necessarily comparable to the subjects interviewed in wave 4. Indeed, the investigators found there were differences in sample characteristics between the waves. To adjust for these differences the investigators performed multivariable logistic regression (column 3). They included in their model those variables that were associated with the wave or with the outcome. The analysis shows that there is a statistically significant decrease of unprotected intercourse at wave 2 and at wave 4.

I will not illustrate all the other statistics listed in Table 6.10 for determining whether there are statistically significant differences between the pre-intervention and post-intervention assessments because the statistics themselves are the same bivariate and multivariable statistics used for any comparison of groups with independent observations. Because performing multivariable analysis with an interval variable with a non-normal distribution is difficult, the easiest recourse is to transform the outcome (e.g. logarithmic transformation) so that it fits assumptions of normality and equal variance. There will be other illustrations of these statistics in Sections 6.5 and 6.6.

6.4 Is the difference between the pre-intervention and the post-intervention assessment of the intervention group statistically greater (lesser) than that seen in the comparison group(s) in a longitudinal cohort study?

Tests for comparing differences in change over time between the intervention group and the comparison group(s) in longitudinal cohorts are shown

Table 6.12. Tests for comparing changes over time between the intervention group and the comparison group(s), longitudinal cohort study.

Measure	Unadjusted comparison between groups (bivariate)	Adjusted comparison between groups (multivariable)
Mean difference between two time points, two groups	Difference between the mean difference of two groups and 95% confidence intervals *t*-test	Multiple linear regression ANOVA ANCOVA
Mean difference between two time points, three or more groups	ANOVA	Multiple linear regression ANOVA ANCOVA
Interval outcome, normal distribution, two or more time points, two or more groups	Repeated measures ANOVA	Repeated measures ANOVA Repeated measures ANCOVA Mixed-effects models
Proportion, two points, two groups	Two-sample generalization of McNemar's test	Conditional logistic regression Mixed-effects models
Proportion, three or more time points, two or more groups	Conditional logistic regression	Conditional logistic regression Mixed-effects models
Difference in time to outcome	Kaplan–Meier	Proportional hazards regression

in Table 6.12. Because there are often baseline differences between the intervention group and the comparison group that require statistical adjustment, I have included multivariable methods as well as bivariate analysis in Table 6.12.

6.4.A Mean difference between two time points, two groups, bivariate analysis

When you have calculated the mean between two time points, an easy way to look for differences between the groups is to calculate the difference between the mean change of the intervention group and the mean change of the comparison group.

Look back at Table 6.3. Using data from the Bright Bodies study, I illustrated the use of mean difference and the 95% confidence intervals to quantify the difference between pre-intervention and post-intervention for a group of overweight children. We saw that there was a significant weight loss among the children who received the intervention. Now, let's see whether the weight loss over time was greater in the intervention group than in the control group.

Table 6.13. Comparison of mean weight loss among overweight children enrolled in Bright Bodies intervention versus the control group.

	Intervention group	Control group	Treatment – Control group
Mean weight change at 6 months	–2.6 kg	5.0 kg	7.6 kg
95% confidence intervals	–4.2 to –0.9 kg	2.9 to 7.2 kg	4.3 to 10.8 kg

Data from: Savoye, M., *et al.* "Effects of a weight management program on body composition and metabolic parameters in overweight children: A randomized controlled trial." *JAMA* **297** (2007): 2697–704.

Column 1 of Table 6.13 shows the loss of weight that occurred in the intervention group in the first 6 months (loss of 2.6 kg), just as in Table 6.3. Column 2 shows that the control group did not lose weight during the same period, but actually gained an average of 5.0 kg. In the last column of the table, you can see the difference between the mean weight loss of the two groups (7.6 kg) that occurred in the first 6 months. The 95% confidence intervals exclude zero, indicating that the difference that occurred between the two groups over time is not likely to be due to chance. The addition of the control group strengthens the inference that the intervention was effective.

Another method of comparing the change in the intervention group to the change in the control group is to use an unpaired *t*-test. For example, Walter and Vaughan evaluated the effectiveness of an AIDS-preventive curriculum on the knowledge, beliefs, self-efficacy, and behavioral risk factors of 9th and 11th grade students.[16]

Looking across the rows of Table 6.14 note that for each measure there is a baseline score, a follow-up score, and the difference between the baseline and follow-up score for both the intervention group and the comparison group. The statistical significance of the *t*-test is reflected in the final column, the *P* value, which is the probability that the observed difference between the change that occurred in the intervention group and the change that occurred in the comparison group could have occurred by chance alone.

> *P* values are highly dependent on sample size and not on clinical importance.

The downside of the use of *P* values as opposed to the mean difference with the 95% confidence intervals (shown in Table 6.13) is that *P* values do not convey the effect size. If your sample is very large (e.g., 10 000 patients) even trivial differences may be statistically significant. Conversely, with a small sample size clinically important differences may not be statistically significant.

---

[16] Walter, H. J. and Vaughan, R. D. "AIDS risk reduction among a multiethnic sample of urban high school students." *JAMA* **270** (1993): 725–30.

Table 6.14. Comparison of changes over time between the intervention and the comparison group.

Outcome variable	Intervention			Comparison			t	P
	Baseline	Follow-up	Difference	Baseline	Follow-up	Difference		
Knowledge	75.6	85.5	9.9	78.8	81.2	2.4	8.9	0.0001
Beliefs susceptibility	2.5	2.1	−0.4	2.5	2.3	−0.2	1.5	0.14
Benefits	3.5	3.8	0.3	3.7	3.8	−0.1	4.7	0.0001
Barriers	4.4	4.5	0.1	4.4	4.4	0	1.2	0.22
Values	5.4	5.5	0.1	5.5	5.5	0	0.7	0.50
Norms	2.8	2.9	0.1	2.8	2.8	0	3.0	0.003
Self-efficacy	3.7	3.9	0.2	3.7	3.8	0.1	2.2	0.03
Behavior risk index	1.5	1.3	−0.2	1.0	1.3	0.3	2.8	0.006

Data from: Walter, H.J., *et al.* "AIDS risk reduction among a multiethnic sample of urban high school students." *JAMA* **270** (1993): 725–30.

6.4.B Mean difference between two time points, three groups, bivariate analysis

Compare the mean difference with three or more groups using ANOVA.

With three or more groups you cannot use a t-test to compare the changes among your groups. Instead, use ANOVA. For example, Tan evaluated the efficacy of phototherapy for reducing neonatal jaundice.[17] As you can see in Table 6.15, the mean decrease in bilirubin in 24 hours differed in the three groups.

The significant P value does not tell you where the difference lies. However, in situations like this, where the P value of the ANOVA is significant, you may then perform pairwise comparisons. Because you will be essentially performing multiple comparisons (formula-fed versus breast-fed infants; formula-fed versus formula- and breast-fed infants; breast-fed versus formula- and breast-fed infants), the P values should be adjusted to be more stringent. One popular method is the Bonferroni correction.[18]

Although the study of infants did not report the Bonferroni correction it is easy to do. It is simply the significance level assuming a single test (usually $P = 0.05$) divided by the number of comparisons performed (in this case three). This then yields a new more stringent P value of 0.017 (0.05/3). The pairwise comparison between breast-fed infants and formula- and breast-fed infants had a P value of 0.007, below the more stringent P value.

---

[17] Tan, K. L. "Decreased response to phototherapy for neonatal jaundice in breast-fed infants." *Arch. Pediatr. Adolesc. Med.* **152** (1998): 1187–90.

[18] Although easy to compute and conceptually appealing the Bonferroni correction can be too conservative, especially with small sample sizes and a large number of pairwise comparisons. For a list and brief description of pairwise tests, see: *Pairwise comparisons in SAS and SPSS* at www.uky.edu/ComputingCenter/SSTARS/www/documentation/MultipleComparisons_3.htm; for a more thorough discussion see: Glantz, S. A. *Primer of Biostatistics* (5th edition). New York: McGraw-Hill, 2002: pp. 89–107.

Table 6.15. Bilirubin decrease with phototherapy.

	Formula-fed infants	Breast-fed infants	Formula- and breast-fed infants	P value
Mean bilirubin decrease, %	18.6	17.1	22.9	0.03

Data from Tan, K. L. "Decreased response to phototheraphy for neonatal jaundice in breast-fed infants." *Arch. Pediatr. Adolesc. Med.* **152** (1998): 1187–90.

> An ANOVA with two groups is the same as an unpaired *t*-test.

You may see articles using ANOVA to compare the difference scores of only two groups. If the difference scores are being compared without adjustment for other factors, then the ANOVA is identical to an unpaired *t*-test.

6.4.C Mean difference between two time points, two or more groups, multivariable analysis

> Use multiple linear regression to adjust for baseline differences when comparing mean changes between groups.

When you are comparing the mean difference among two or more different groups, you may need to adjust for baseline differences between the groups. The simplest method for adjusting for baseline differences is multiple linear regression. For example, in the study (above) evaluating the effectiveness of an AIDS-preventive intervention, the investigators used multiple linear regression to adjust their data for baseline differences.

In their linear regression model the outcome was the follow-up score, and the independent variables were the intervention group, the baseline score, age, gender, and race/ethnicity. The standardized regression coefficients shown in Table 6.16 represent the adjusted change in the outcome variable that is due to the intervention. All the changes were statistically significant except that for the variable "values."

If you have more than two groups, you will need to create multiple dichotomous variables to represent the groups. The number of variables you will need will be 1 less than the number of groups you have. For example, if you have three groups A, B and C, you will create two variables: group A (yes/no) and group B (yes/no) and enter them into the model as independent variables.[19]

You can also adjust for baseline differences using ANOVA or an ANCOVA. With ANOVA you can include baseline variables that are dichotomous or nominal such as sex and ethnicity. When you need to adjust for interval covariates instead of, or in addition to, dichotomous or nominal variables use analysis of covariance (ANCOVA).

[19] For more on creating multiple dichotomous variables see Katz, M. H. *Multivariable Analysis: A Practical Guide for Clinicians* (2nd edition). Cambridge: Cambridge University Press: pp. 35–7.

Table 6.16. Standardized linear regression coefficients for intervention effect on outcome variables.

Outcome variable	Standardized coefficients*	P value
Knowledge	0.25	<0.001
Beliefs		
Susceptibility	−0.08	<0.01
Benefits	0.08	<0.01
Barriers	0.05	<0.05
Values	0.03	NS
Norms	0.09	<0.01
Self-efficacy	0.07	<0.01
Behavior risk index	−0.10	<0.01

*Coefficients are adjusted for age, gender, race/ethnicity, and baseline value on scale. Data from: Walter, H.J., *et al.* "AIDS risk reduction among a multiethnic sample of urban high school students." *JAMA* **270** (1993): 725–30.

6.4.D Interval outcome, two or more time points, two or more groups

> With interval outcomes, two or more groups, and two or more time points, use repeated measures ANOVA.

When you are comparing two or more groups, use repeated measures ANOVA to compare changes across two or more time points.

Repeated measures ANOVA is an extension of ANOVA that can be used to compare changes over time at multiple points with two or more groups. For example, in the study by Belfort and colleagues evaluating the effectiveness of the medication pioglitazone (mentioned above) in treating non-alcoholic steatohepatitis, the researchers compared the effect of pioglitazone to placebo on several parameters (Table 6.17). The *P* values shown under the headings pioglitazone and placebo are based on a paired *t*-test. This is a **within-group** comparison (i.e., is there a statistically significant change between the before and after treatment assessment). It is exactly the same test as discussed in Section 6.2.A.

The *P* value in Table 6.17 for pioglitazone versus placebo (final column) is based on a repeated measures analysis of variance. It answers the statistical question: is the change over time different for the subjects who received pioglitazone than for those who received placebo? This is a **between-group** comparison, and the answer in this case is that the difference between the two assessments is greater in the pioglitazone group than in the placebo group.

> If an intervention really works then the change in the intervention group should be significantly larger than the change in the control group.

In Section 6.2 we considered an intervention to have worked if there was a significant difference between the pre-intervention and the post-intervention assessments. However, with a control group we only conclude that an intervention works when the change in the intervention group is significantly larger than the change in the control group.

If you have any doubt that there must be a significantly larger change in the intervention group than in the control group to conclude that the intervention

Table 6.17. Comparison of pioglitazone to placebo for the treatment of non-alcoholic steatohepatitis.

Variable	Pioglitazone ($n = 26$)			Placebo ($n = 21$)			P value (pioglitazone vs. placebo)
	Before treatment	After treatment	P value	Before treatment	After treatment	P value	
Body-mass index	33.5	34.6	<0.001	32.9	32.7	0.62	0.005
Weight (kg)	93.7	96.2	<0.001	90.2	89.7	0.53	0.003
Body fat (%)	33.7	35.2	<0.01	35.7	34.9	0.78	0.005
Fasting plasma glucose (mg/dl)	119	99	0.004	115	116	0.75	0.011
Glycated hemoglobin (%)	6.2	5.5	<0.001	6.2	6.1	0.73	0.008

Data from Belfort, R., *et al.* "A placebo-controlled trial of pioglitazone in subjects with nonalcoholic steatohepatitis." *N. Engl. J. Med.* **355** (2006): 2297–307.

works, consider the following situation. An investigator evaluates the effectiveness of an intervention to decrease symptoms of depression; a control group is included. The investigator finds that over time both groups report decreased symptoms of depression, but the within-group improvement for the intervention arm is just under the $P < 0.05$ threshold, while the within-group improvement for the control group is just over the threshold. In a case such as this, the between-group comparison will not be statistically significant and it is likely that some factor other than the intervention resulted in improvement in both groups.

A study by Anderson and colleagues illustrates the use of repeated measures analysis of variance for an outcome measured at multiple points in time. The investigators randomized obese women to two different interventions: diet plus aerobic exercise or diet plus lifestyle activity. As you can see in Figure 6.1, both groups lost weight, but there was no significant difference between the two groups in terms of how much weight was lost.[20]

6.4.E Interval outcome, two or more time points, two or more groups, multivariable analysis

> It is possible to adjust for dichotomous or nominal variables within a repeated measures ANOVA.

The technique repeated measures ANOVA allows adjustment for baseline variables if the variable is dichotomous or nominal. If the baseline variable is interval use repeated measures ANCOVA. For example, Lautenschlager and colleagues evaluated the impact of a physical activity program on older adults with memory problems.[21] Subjects were randomized to an activity group or to usual care. A variety of cognitive indices were measured at baseline,

[20] Andersen, R. E., Waddan, T. A., Bartlett, S. J., Zemel, B., Verde, T. J., and Franckowiak, S. C. "Effects of lifestyle activity vs structured aerobic exercise on obese women: A randomized trial." *JAMA* **281** (1999): 335–40.

[21] Lautenschlager, N. T., Cox, K. L., Flicker, L., *et al.* "Effect of physical activity on cognitive function in older adults at risk for Alzheimer disease." *JAMA* **300** (2008): 1027–37.

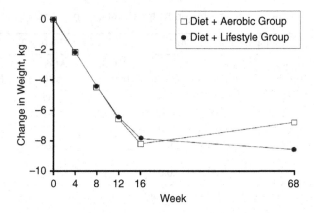

Figure 6.1

Mean change in body weight over time among women randomized to two different interventions. Reprinted with permission from Andersen, R.E., *et al.* "Effects of lifestyle activity vs structured aerobic exercise on obese women: A randomized trial." *JAMA* **281** (1999): 335–40. Copyright © 1999 American Medical Association. All rights reserved.

6 months, 12 months, and 18 months. The investigators used repeated measures ANCOVA so that they could assess changes over time adjusted for both interval variables (e.g., age, premorbid IQ) and categorical variables (e.g., sex, marital status). They found that exercise was associated with a modest improvement in cognition.

Repeated measures ANOVA and repeated measures ANCOVA have several weaknesses. For example, there must be an equal number of observations per subject and fixed periods of time between observations. Also, repeated measures ANOVA and repeated measures ANCOVA assume sphericity. In a longitudinal study sphericity means that the correlation between any two measurements at different time points is the same and that within subjects there is equal variance of measurements. When you have three or more measurements this assumption is often not met. For these reasons, investigators are increasingly using mixed-effects models or generalized estimating equations when comparing changes over time in an interval variable over time. Unfortunately, these procedures are beyond the scope of this book.[22]

> To adjust for both interval and categorical variables use repeated measures analysis of covariance (ANCOVA).

[22] Twisk, J. W. R. *Applied Longitudinal Data Analysis for Epidemiology: A Practical Guide.* Cambridge: Cambridge University Press, 2003: pp. 62–95; Diggle, P. J., Heagerty, P., Liang K.-Y., *et al. Analysis of Longitudinal Data* (2nd edition). Oxford: Oxford University Press, 2002: pp. 128–30, 138–40; Davis, C. S. *Statistical Methods for the Analysis of Repeated Measurements.* New York: Springer-Verlag, 2003: pp. 293, 295–313; Katz, M. H. *Multivariable Analysis: A Practical Guide for Clinicians.* Cambridge: Cambridge University Press, 2006: pp. 164–71.

Table 6.18. Impact of a community mobilization in reducing high-risk sex among young gay men.

	Group	Pre-intervention %	Post-intervention %	Pre- to post-intervention difference, %	P (within group)	P (intervention vs. control)
Unprotected anal intercourse in prior 2 months	Intervention	41.0	30.0	−11.0	<0.05	P <0.03
	Control	38.6	39.8	1.2	NS	

NS = non-significant.

Data from Kegeles, S. M., Hays, R. B., and Coates, T. J. "The Mpowerment project: A community-level HIV prevention intervention for young gay men." *Am. J. Public Health* **86** (1996): 1129–36.

6.4.F Dichotomous outcome, two or more time points, two or more groups, bivariate and multivariable

You will remember from Section 6.2.C that McNemar's test is used to assess the change occurring between two time points (e.g., pre-intervention and post-intervention) in one sample when you have a dichotomous variable. When you have two samples, the difference can be compared using a two-sample generalization of McNemar's test. For example, Kegeles and colleagues developed and implemented a community-level HIV-prevention program for young gay men in a mid-sized community.[23] Young men in the intervention community were surveyed before and after the intervention and young men in a comparison community were surveyed at two similar times. The intervention was successful at decreasing high-risk behavior in the intervention community compared to the comparison community based on the two-sample generalization of McNemar's test (Table 6.18).

In situations where you have more than two time points or when you need to adjust for baseline differences, you will not be able to use the two-sample generalization of McNemar's test. Instead, one option is to use conditional logistic regression analysis. Conditional logistic regression, like standard logistic regression, is used with dichotomous outcomes, but unlike standard logistic regression it can incorporate multiple observations of the same subject.

However, as is true of the family of ANOVA procedures, conditional logistic regression can only be used if there are the same number of observations at each time point. Mixed-effects models and generalized estimating equations are more flexible in that they allow for multiple data points of the same persons and differences in the numbers of observations among the subjects (see footnote 22 above).

[23] Kegeles, S. M., Hays, R. B., and Coates, T. J. "The Mpowerment project: A community-level HIV prevention intervention for young gay men." *Am. J. Public Health* **86** (1996): 1129–36.

6.4.G Comparison of time to outcome, two or more groups, bivariate and multivariable

We are often interested in whether an intervention affects time to outcome (e.g., time to death, time to recurrence of cancer). To determine time to outcome we use survival analyses, a group of procedures that incorporate time into the analysis. Survival curves are used to describe the proportion of persons experiencing an event over a period of time. The most common method of calculating a survival curve is the Kaplan–Meier method. To determine whether an intervention affects time to outcome we can compare the Kaplan–Meier curves of two or more groups using the log-rank statistic.

For example, Johnson and colleagues used Kaplan–Meier curves to assess the efficacy of topiramate for treating alcohol dependence.[24] They found that those subjects randomized to topiramate had shorter times to continuous abstinence than those who received placebo (Figure 6.2). The difference between the two curves was statistically significant (*P* value of log-rank test <0.001).

An important feature of survival curves, and of survival analyses generally, is that the technique enables us to incorporate subjects who have been lost to follow-up, withdrawn from the study without allowing themselves to be followed, or have an outcome that precludes them from being assessed for the outcome of interest (e.g., a subject enrolled in a study of time to cancer dies in a car accident). The feature is called censoring and it enables us to include subjects with different lengths of follow-up.[25]

For example, in the study of topiramate versus placebo, 179 subjects were enrolled in the topiramate arm and 185 were enrolled in the placebo arm. However, only 112 subjects in the topiramate arm and 144 subjects in the placebo arm actually finished the trial. Other subjects experienced a limiting side effect, withdrew, were lost to follow-up or did not complete the trial for other reasons. With censoring, subjects contribute their experience until the time that they leave the study. In this way, vital observation time is not lost, as would occur if all subjects who did not complete a trial were excluded.

The numbers under the survival curve of Figure 6.2 indicate the number of people who are at risk for the outcome in the next period of time. Conversely, those people who had a limiting side effect, withdrew, were lost to follow-up, did not complete the study for some other reason, or had already experienced the outcome of interest (abstinence) are no longer counted. That's the reason as time progresses fewer and fewer people are shown in the legend to be at risk for

> Survival analyses can incorporate subjects who have been lost to follow-up, withdrawn from the study, or have an outcome that precludes them from being assessed for the outcome of interest.

> Censoring enables us to include subjects with different lengths of follow-up.

> **TIP**
> Always include a legend under a survival curve showing the number of subjects at risk in the next time period.

---

[24] Johnson, B. A., Rosenthal, N., Capece, J. A., *et al.* "Topiramate for treating alcohol dependence: A randomized controlled trial." *JAMA* **298** (2007): 1641–51.

[25] For more on censoring, including the underlying assumptions of censoring and how to test whether your data fulfill these assumptions see Katz, M. H. *Study Design and Statistical Analysis: A Practical Guide for Clinicians*. Cambridge: Cambridge University Press, 2006: pp. 61–4.

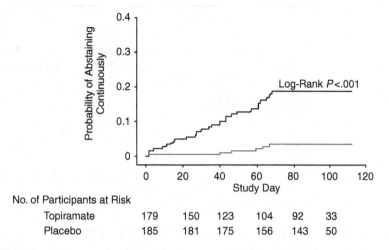

No. of Participants at Risk

Topiramate	179	150	123	104	92	33
Placebo	185	181	175	156	143	50

Figure 6.2   Kaplan–Meier curves comparing time to continuous abstinence among persons on topiramate and those on placebo. Reprinted with permission from Johnson, B.A., *et al.* "Topiramate for treating alcohol dependence: A randomized controlled trial." *JAMA* **298** (2007): 1641–51. Copyright © 2007 American Medical Association. All rights reserved.

the outcome. Investigators should always show the numbers of subjects at risk in the legend of their Kaplan–Meier curves otherwise the reader cannot assess the validity of the results; as the sample size shrinks the estimates of percentage outcome in the next period of time become less certain.

Often when comparing the time to outcome of different groups we will want to adjust for baseline differences. For example, in Section 3.4 I cited a study by Hannan and colleagues as an example of using a procedure database to evaluate an intervention.

In that study the investigators assessed how well drug-eluting stents (a new technology) worked compared to coronary artery bypass grafting (CABG), among persons with multivessel coronary artery disease. Since patients were identified through two registries and were not randomized into two groups, there were significant differences between patients in the two groups. Patients undergoing CABG were older, more likely to be male, to be non-Hispanic, to be white, to have lower ejection fractions, to have had previous myocardial infarctions, to have other coexisting conditions, and to have three-vessel disease. To adjust for these differences, the investigators used proportional hazards analysis. They found that patients who received a CABG had a lower risk of death and myocardial infarction than patients who received a drug-eluting stent (Table 6.19). Despite the lack of randomization the results of the study have been broadly accepted and CABG remains the treatment of choice for persons with multivessel disease.

Table 6.19. Hazard ratios for death and for death or myocardial infarction after CABG and after treatment with a drug-eluting stent, according to number of diseased vessels.*

Variable	Death		Death or myocardial infarction	
	Adjusted relative hazard* (95% CI)	P value	Adjusted relative hazard* (95% CI)	P value
Three diseased vessels				
With or without proximal LAD artery				
CABG	0.80 (0.65–0.97)	0.03	0.75 (0.63–0.89)	<0.001
Stent	Reference		Reference	
With proximal LAD artery				
CABG	0.79 (0.61–1.02)	0.07	0.77 (0.61–0.96)	0.02
Stent	Reference		Reference	
Without proximal LAD artery				
CABG	0.79 (0.58–1.09)	0.15	0.69 (0.53–0.91)	0.008
Stent	Reference		Reference	
Two diseased vessels				
With or without proximal LAD artery				
CABG	0.71 (0.57–0.89)	0.003	0.71 (0.59–0.87)	<0.001
Stent	Reference		Reference	
With proximal LAD artery				
CABG	0.71 (0.53–0.96)	0.02	0.72 (0.56–0.93)	0.01
Stent	Reference		Reference	
Without proximal LAD artery				
CABG	0.69 (0.48–0.98)	0.04	0.71 (0.52–0.96)	0.03
Stent	Reference		Reference	

CABG denotes coronary-artery bypass grafting, and LAD left anterior descending.
* Relative hazards are adjusted for age, sex; ejection fraction; hemodynamic state; history or no history of myocardial infarction before procedure; presence or absence of cerebrovascular disease, peripheral arterial disease, congestive heart failure, chronic obstructive pulmonary disease, diabetes, and renal failure; and involvement of the proximal LAD artery.
Data from Hannan, E. L., *et al.* "Drug-eluting stents vs. coronary-artery bypass grafting in multivessel coronary artery disease." *N. Engl. J. Med.* **358** (2008): 331–41.

Table 6.20. Multivariable techniques for assessing whether the change from baseline to follow-up is greater (less) in the intervention group than in the comparison group.

Outcome measure	Multivariable analysis
Dichotomous	Multiple logistic regression
Interval, normal distribution	Multiple linear regression
	ANOVA
	ANCOVA
Interval, non-normal distribution	–*
Ordinal	Proportional odds regression
Time to outcome	Proportional hazards (Cox) analysis

* Attempt to transform the outcome variable so that it fits the assumptions of normality and equal variance.

6.5 Is the difference between the pre-intervention and the post-intervention assessment of the intervention group statistically greater (lesser) than that seen in the comparison group(s) in a serial cross-sectional study?

As with cohort studies, serial cross-sectional studies are also strengthened by having a comparison group. For serial cross-sectional studies with a control group multivariable analysis will almost always be necessary because there will be differences within groups and between groups. Therefore, I have shown only multivariable techniques for this type of study design (Table 6.20). As you can see the appropriate multivariable technique depends on the type of outcome measure you have.

Beyond the standard multivariable analyses listed in Table 6.20, generalized estimating equations and mixed-effects models can also be used to answer whether the change is greater in the intervention group than in the comparison group. These models are very flexible and can also incorporate linked observations.

To illustrate the statistical analysis of serial cross-sectional data with a control group, let's look at a study by Snyder and Anderson. The investigators assessed whether participation in a quality improvement organization improved the care of Medicare beneficiaries.[26] They abstracted the medical records of one group of patients at baseline and the medical records of a different set of patients at follow-up; they assessed improvement on 15 quality indicators that were the focus of the quality improvement organizations during the period between the baseline and follow-up surveys.

Results for two of the 15 indicators are shown in Table 6.21. The *P* values for the (within-group) differences between the pre-intervention and post-intervention are based on chi-squared analyses, just as you would do if you were performing a serial cross-sectional study without a comparison group (Section 6.3).

Answering the question of whether the change is greater in the intervention group than in the comparison group will require multivariable analysis because we will need to adjust for differences in the samples. The outcome for this study is performance of the quality indicator (yes/no). Because the outcome is dichotomous the authors used multiple logistic regression. The independent variables were participation in the quality improvement organization (yes/no), period (baseline/follow-up), and an interaction between participation in the quality improvement program and period. The interaction tells you whether participating hospitals during the study period improved more or less than nonparticipating hospitals during the study period. In these models the

---

[26] Snyder, C. and Anderson, G. "Do quality improvement organizations improve the quality of hospital care for Medicare beneficiaries." *JAMA* **293** (2005): 2900–7.

Table 6.21. Comparison of changes on two quality indicators among hospitals that did or did not participate in quality improvement organization.

	Participated in quality improvement organization				Did not participate in quality improvement organization				Intervention effect		
	Baseline	Follow-up	Change	P value	Baseline	Follow-up	Change	P value	Difference in change	Adjusted odds ratio*	P value
Aspirin prescribed at discharge following heart attack	85.3	88.0	2.7	0.09	83.6	87.7	4.1	0.13	1.4	0.95 (0.56–1.61)	0.85
Patient screened for or given pneumococcal vaccine	15.5	40.9	25.4	<0.0001	8.4	17.1	8.7	<0.0001	16.7	1.58 (1.15–2.18)	0.005

* Odds ratios are adjusted for patient age, sex, and race and hospital bed size and profit status.

Data from Snyder, C., and Andersow, G. "Do quality improvement organizations improve the quality of hospital care for medicaid beneficiaries?" *JAMA* **293** (2005): 2900–7.

investigators adjusted for patient age, sex, and race, and hospital bed size and profit status.

The results of the multiple logistic regression analysis appear in the final column. There was no change in the likelihood of aspirin prescription, but patients in participating hospitals were more likely to be screened or given pneumococcal vaccine.

Because multiple patients were seen in the same hospital, the authors supplemented their main analysis, by performing generalized estimating equations to adjust for the effect of clustering within hospitals. Results were similar so the investigators only reported the results from the more conventional multiple logistic regression analysis.

6.6 Is the post-intervention assessment of the intervention group significantly different than the corresponding assessment of the comparison group?

As discussed in Section 1.2.C, there are times when no pre-intervention measure is available to evaluate an intervention. Instead, an intervention group is compared to a comparison group on a specific outcome. The bivariate and multivariable statistics for comparing a post-intervention assessment of an intervention group to the corresponding assessment of the control group are shown in Table 6.22. As was true of the other statistics listed in this chapter, the choice of statistic depends on the nature of the outcome variable.

You will note that these are the same statistics for comparing pre-intervention versus post-intervention measures with serial cross-sectional data (Section 6.3). This is because in both cases the observations are unlinked.

To demonstrate differences between the group that received the intervention and the control group you will generally need to use multivariable statistics because there will likely be baseline differences between the groups (unless there was a natural randomization that formed the groups – an unlikely circumstance).

For example, Tseng and colleagues evaluated whether Medicare drug benefit caps affected the ability of seniors to obtain their medication.[27] After the drug caps were implemented, the investigators surveyed two groups of seniors: those who had a $750 or $1200 yearly cap and had exceeded it in the prior year (intervention group) and those who had a $2000 cap which they had not exceeded

---

[27] Tseng C.-W., Brook, R. H., Keeler, E., Steers, W. N., and Mangione, C. M. "Cost-lowering strategies used by Medicare beneficiaries who exceed drug benefit caps and have a gap in drug coverage." *JAMA* **292** (2004): 952–60.

Table 6.22. Tests for comparing the outcome of an intervention group to a comparison group(s).

Outcome measure	Two groups bivariate	Three or more groups bivariate	Multivariable analysis
Dichotomous	Chi-squared Fisher's exact Odds ratio	Chi-squared	Multiple logistic regression
Interval, normal distribution	t-test	ANOVA	Multiple linear regression ANOVA ANCOVA
Interval, non-normal distribution	Mann–Whitney test	Kruskal–Wallis test	*–
Ordinal	Mann–Whitney test	Kruskal–Wallis test	Proportional odds regression

*Attempt to transform the outcome variable so that it fits the assumptions of normality and equal variance.

(control group) – since they had not exceeded it we can assume that they were essentially unaffected by the cap.

The investigators performed a stratified sample of potential controls to identify controls that were similar in age and monthly drug expenditures to those affected by the intervention. Nonetheless, there were significant differences between the intervention and the control group. Controls were more likely to be women, less likely to be married, had lower household income, higher rates of hypertension and emphysema, and a higher mean number of health conditions.

As you can see in Table 6.23, seniors in the intervention group were more likely to adopt strategies to decrease their medication usage, including taking less medication than prescribed, switching medications, using medication samples, calling pharmacies to find the best price, and receiving a discount for being over 65 years. The percentages and the P values were based on multiple logistic regression analysis adjusting for age, sex, education, ethnicity, household income, health status, functional limitations, number of health problems, type of survey, and whether income data were present.

Although the analyses were adjusted for differences between participants in the intervention group and those in the control group, there remains the possibility that underlying differences between these groups explain the differences in their strategies to decrease medication usage. The fact that the different caps were offered in different counties meant that individuals did not self-select to the different caps (which would have made the study design much more problematic) but the baseline characteristics tell us that the participants in the different counties were different.

This problem could have been eliminated if the caps could have been randomized, but randomizing types of insurance coverage for government

Table 6.23. Adjusted percentages of elders who used strategies to lower medication costs.

	Adjusted percentages		
	Intervention participants: exceeded $750 or $1200 cap ($n = 665$)	Control participants: did not exceed $2000 cap ($n = 643$)	P value*
Medication strategies for decreasing costs that involve decreasing use			
Used less medication than was prescribed or less than desired (e.g., skipped dose)	18	10	<0.001
Stopped a medication	8	8	0.86
Did not fill a prescription for a new medication (i.e., did not start a new medication)	6	5	0.39
Adopted at least 1 strategy above that decreased medication use	24	16	<0.001
Strategies for decreasing cost that may or may not involve decreasing use			
Switched medications	15	9	0.002
Received free medication samples	34	27	0.006
Took someone else's medication	2	1	0.26
Called pharmacies to find the best price	46	29	<0.001
Strategies for obtaining discounts			
Received discount for being age >65 yr	12	7	0.003
Received discount for being in Medicare	10	7	0.13
Received discount from a pharmaceutical company	2	1	0.11
Used mail order	63	62	0.64
Bought medications outside the United States	3	3	0.92

* The adjusted difference is based on multivariate logistic regression including age, sex, education, ethnicity, annual household income, general health status, functional limitations in instrumental activities of daily living, number of health problems, written vs. telephone survey, and whether or not participants had income data as covariates. Data from Tseng, C.-W., Brook, R.H., Keeler, E., Steers, W.N., and Mangione, C.M. "Cost-lowering strategies used by Medicare beneficiaries who exceed drug benefit caps and have a gap in drug coverage." *JAMA* **292** (2004): 952–60.

programs is not a very feasible study design. A pre-intervention measure of the same strategies would have made this study stronger – even stronger would have been evidence that seniors actually stopped taking medicines that they were taking prior to the caps. However, in the real world of health policy, this study makes a compelling case that cost caps change the behavior of seniors.

As discussed in Section 1.2.C, case-control studies can be used to assess whether an intervention has been successful in cases where there is no pre-intervention measurement. The statistics used to analyze case-control studies are the same as those listed in Table 6.21, as long as the cases and controls are not one-to-one matched.[28] For example, Werler and colleagues used a case-control design to demonstrate that folic acid was effective in reducing neural tube defects. They identified 436 mothers with a baby born with a neural tube defect (cases) and 2615 mothers with a baby born with a malformation other than neural tube (controls). They asked the mothers about their consumption of folic acid-containing supplements in the periconceptual period. Eight percent of the cases versus 13% of the controls had taken daily folic acid in the preconceptual period, indicating that folic acid was associated with a significant reduction in the odds of having a neural tube defect (OR = 0.57, 95% CI = 0.4–0.8).[29]

To minimize the effect of confounding, the investigators also performed multiple logistic regression adjusting for all those variables that altered the crude odds ratio. With adjustment, daily folic acid was still associated with decreased odds of a neural tube defect. As with any study that relies on subjects reporting prior events, there is the possibility that there was differential reporting of folic acid use. The investigators addressed differential reporting by limiting their analysis to women who had not heard of the hypothesis that folic acid reduced birth defects. In this subgroup, preconceptual use of folic acid was still associated with significantly reduced neural tube defects (multivariable OR = 0.4, 95% CI = 0.2–0.6).

Of course, the chance that there were other important differences between the cases and controls on recall or other issues remains. Nonetheless, when prospective studies were performed, folic acid was found to reduce neural tube defects.[30] This case-control study helped to spark further research and ultimately contributed to the recommendation that all women who may become pregnant in the near future take folic acid.

---

[28] For more on bivariate analysis of matched data see Katz, M. H. *Study Design and Statistical Analysis: A Practical Guide for Clinicians*. Cambridge: Cambridge University Press, 1996: pp. 116–9. For multivariable analysis of matched data see Katz, M. H. *Multivariable Analysis: A Practical Guide for Clinicians*. Cambridge: Cambridge University Press, 1996: pp. 158–78.

[29] If you look at the original article the authors report relative risk but state that they estimated it from the odds ratio. I couldn't reproduce their crude odds ratio exactly so the one I report (calculated from the raw data with www.openepi.com) is slightly different from what is in the reported article. It is true that when the exposure (in this case taking folic acid) is uncommon (<15%), the odds ratio approximates the relative risk.

[30] Berry, R. J., Li, Z., Erickson, J. D., *et al.* "Prevention of neural-tube defects with folic acid in China." *N. Engl. J. Med.* **341** (1999): 1485–90.

Methods for adjusting for baseline differences between treatment groups

7.1 How do I adjust for baseline differences between persons who receive the intervention and those who don't?

In Section 5.3, I illustrated how baseline differences between treatment groups could confound the results of a study. The specific example was influenza vaccination among the elderly. Because physicians tended to immunize the sickest patients, it appeared that vaccination was associated with **higher** rates of hospitalization for respiratory conditions. However, once the investigators used multivariable analysis to adjust for confounders, elders who were vaccinated were **less** likely to have been hospitalized due to respiratory conditions than elders who were not vaccinated.

Although multivariable analysis is a powerful tool for adjusting for baseline differences, at times, especially with nonrandomized studies, it is not sufficient. In such situations, two advanced methods are increasingly being used for achieving comparable groups: propensity score analysis and instrumental variable analysis. Because these methods require multivariable analysis, I explain their advantages and disadvantages compared to performing multivariable analysis alone, as well as compared to each other (Table 7.1).

7.2 What are propensity scores? How are they calculated?

Propensity scores are used to adjust for baseline differences between groups.

Propensity scores are a statistical method for adjusting for baseline differences between study groups.

The use of propensity scores is a two-part process: (1) the development of the score and (2) the use of the score for adjusting for baseline differences.

To calculate a propensity score first identify those variables that influence study group membership.

Propensity scores are calculations of the probability of a subject being in a particular group, conditional upon that subject's values on variables that influence group membership. To calculate the propensity score first identify those variables that influence study group membership (e.g., demographic characteristics, disease severity).

Table 7.1. Comparison of multivariable analysis, propensity-score analysis, and instrumental variable analysis for adjusting for baseline differences in study groups.

	Advantages	Disadvantages
Multivariable analysis alone	Backbone of all methods for adjusting for baseline differences. It is less frightening to non-statistically inclined readers than propensity-score and instrumental variable analyses.	Does not work well if there are many baseline differences relative to the number of outcomes in the study. Adjusting for a large number of variables may result in a misspecified model and may make it more difficult to perform diagnostic checks on the model. If the distribution of confounders does not sufficiently overlap between the groups, effect estimates are based on extrapolation and may be unreliable. Cannot adjust for unmeasured confounders.
Propensity-score analysis	Can be used in situations where there are many baseline differences and relatively few outcomes, as long as the sample is relatively evenly split among the study groups. Can make unlimited attempts at balancing covariates without worrying about biasing your analysis. Makes no assumption about the relationship of the baseline characteristic and the outcome.	If group membership is not evenly split, there may not be a large enough sample size to develop valid propensity scores. There must be sufficient overlap between the groups for the technique to work. If you use propensity scores to match, your matched samples may no longer be representative of the underlying population. Cannot adjust for unmeasured confounders.
Instrumental variable analysis	Only method that can account for unmeasured confounders. Good for policy-level analyses.	Not always possible to identify an instrumental variable. Decreases precision of estimate of effect. Results are generalizable only to patients for whom the instrument determined whether they received the intervention (the "marginal" patient). Not appropriate for estimating the benefit of an intervention for an individual.

The variables that influence group membership are then entered into a logistic model (assuming two groups) estimating the likelihood of being in a particular group. A logistic model will yield a propensity score for each subject ranging from 0 to 1; the score is the estimated probability of being in one group versus the other, conditional on a weighted score of that subject's values on the set of variables used to create the score.

To understand the strength of propensity scores, consider two subjects with identical propensity scores, one who received the intervention and one who did not. If we assume that the propensity score is based on all those factors that

Propensity scores are the probability of a subject being in a particular group, conditional on that subject's values on those variables thought to influence group membership.

If two subjects have the same propensity score and we have not missed any confounders, then group assignment can be thought of as random.

would affect the likelihood of receiving an intervention, then we can consider the assignment of the cases to be essentially random.[1]

Of course, even if your propensity score is based on all of the factors known to influence group assignment, there remains the possibility that there are unknown confounders. If you could include these unknown confounders, they would change the propensity score. Therefore, two subjects with the same propensity score may not have the same likelihood of being in either group.[2]

Gum and colleagues used propensity scores to assess whether aspirin use decreased mortality among patients suspected of coronary artery disease.[3] Subjects were drawn from consecutive adult patients undergoing stress echocardiography at a single center. Of 6174 patients meeting the eligibility criteria of the study, 2310 (37%) were taking aspirin and 3864 (63%) were not.

As you can see in Table 7.2 there were numerous baseline differences between patients taking aspirin and those not taking aspirin. In particular, those patients taking aspirin are older and sicker (more likely to be diabetic, hypertensive, have prior coronary artery disease, etc.) and would therefore be expected to have higher mortality. Therefore a comparison of the two groups would not be valid unless the analysis was adjusted to make the groups more comparable.

To create comparable groups, the investigators created propensity scores for each subject using logistic regression. The outcome for the model (dependent variable) was whether or not the patient received aspirin. The model included 34 baseline characteristics (independent variables), some of which are included in Table 7.2. This resulted in a score for each patient, ranging from 0.03 to 0.98, representing the probability that a patient would be using aspirin.

Propensity scores are calculated without regard to outcome.

Note that the propensity score is calculated without regard to the outcome (in the case of this study the outcome was mortality). This leads to an important advantage of propensity scores. In comparison to the traditional approach of adjusting for baseline differences by including them in a multivariable model, the propensity score can be calculated without consideration of the outcome variable. This means that it is possible to experiment with inclusion of different combinations of variables in the propensity score without risking biasing your model by choosing variables based on how they affect your estimate of outcome.

[1] Rubin, D. B. "Estimating causal effects from large data sets using propensity scores." *Ann. Intern. Med.* **127** (1997): 757–63.

[2] D'Agostino, R. B. "Propensity score methods for bias reduction in the comparison of a treatment to a non-randomized control group." *Statist. Med.* **17** (1998): 2265–81.

[3] Gum, P. A., Thamilarasan, M., Watanabe, J., Blackstone, E. H., and Lauer, M. S. "Aspirin use and all-cause mortality among patients being evaluated for known or suspected coronary artery disease: A propensity analysis." *JAMA* **286** (2001): 1187–94.

Table 7.2. Baseline characteristics of aspirin and non-aspirin users.

	Aspirin (*n* = 2310)	No aspirin (*n* = 3864)	*P* value
Demographics			
Age, mean (SD), yr	62 (11)	56 (12)	<0.001
Men, no. (%)	1779 (77)	2167 (56)	<0.001
Clinical history			
Diabetes, no. (%)	388 (17)	432 (11)	<0.001
Hypertension, no. (%)	1224 (53)	1569 (41)	<0.001
Tobacco use, no. (%)	234 (10)	500 (13)	0.001
Prior coronary artery disease, no. (%)	1609 (70)	778 (20)	<0.001
Prior coronary artery bypass graft, no. (%)	689 (30)	240 (6)	<0.001
Prior percutaneous coronary interv., no. (%)	667 (29)	148 (4)	<0.001
Prior Q-wave MI, no. (%)	369 (16)	285 (7)	<0.001
Atrial fibrillation, no. (%)	27 (1)	55 (1)	0.04
Congestive heart failure, no. (%)	127 (6)	178 (5)	0.12
Medication use			
Digoxin use, no. (%)	171 (7)	216 (6)	0.004
β-Blocker use, no. (%)	811 (35)	550 (14)	<0.001
Diltiazem/verapamil use, no. (%)	452 (20)	405 (10)	<0.001
Nifedipine use, no. (%)	261 (11)	283 (7)	<0.001
Lipid-lowering therapy, no. (%)	775 (34)	380 (10)	<0.001
ACE inhibitor use, no. (%)	349 (15)	441 (11)	<0.001
Cardiovascular assessment and exercise capacity			
Body mass index, mean (SD), kg/m^2	29 (5)	30 (7)	<0.001
Ejection fraction, mean (SD), %	50 (9)	53 (7)	<0.001
Resting heart rate, mean (SD), beats/min	74 (13)	79 (14)	<0.001
Systolic blood pressure, mean (SD), mmHg	141 (21)	138 (20)	<0.001
Diastolic blood pressure, mean (SD), mmHg	85 (11)	86 (11)	0.04
Purpose of test to evaluate chest pain, no. (%)	300 (13)	468 (12)	0.31
Mayo Risk Index >1, no. (%)	2021 (87)	2517 (65)	<0.001
Peak exercise capacity, mean (SD), METs			
Men	8.6 (2.4)	9.1 (2.6)	<0.001
Women	6.6 (2.0)	7.3 (2.1)	<0.001
Heart rate recovery, mean (SD), beats/min	28 (11)	30 (12)	<0.001
Ischemic ECG charges with stress, no. (%)	430 (24)	457 (14)	<0.001
Ejection fraction < 40%, no. (%)	321 (14)	226 (6)	<0.001
Stress-induced ischemia on echo, no. (%)	495 (21)	436 (11)	<0.001
Fair or poor physical fitness, no. (%)	714 (31)	1248 (38)	0.26

Data from: Gum, P. A., *et al.* "Aspirin use and all-cause mortality among patients being evaluated for known or suspected coronary artery disease: A propensity analysis." *JAMA* **286** (2001): 1187–94.

> Propensity scores can be used in four different ways: matching, stratification, as a covariate, and as a method for weighting observations.

Once the propensity score is created, it can be used to adjust for baseline differences in four different ways: matching, stratification, as a covariate in a multivariable analysis, and as a method for weighting observations. These different methods are discussed in Sections 7.5.A–E. However, first let's answer two important questions with regard to how to calculate propensity scores: what variables to include in a propensity score and how to assess the adequacy of propensity scores.

7.3 Which variables should be included in a propensity score?

There is some controversy over which variables to include in creating a propensity score. Should you include: (1) all those variables that are associated with treatment assignment; (2) all those variables that are associated with the outcome; (3) only those variables that are associated with treatment and outcome (true confounders)?[4]

Based on the discussion of confounding (Section 5.3) it might seem sufficient to include only those variables that are associated with both the treatment and the outcome (choice #3 above). After all, if a variable is not a confounder then its inclusion in a propensity score is not likely to improve the adjustment for differences between the two groups. Also by limiting the variables in the score to the confounders (1) the efficiency of the model creating the score will increase and (2) it will be easier to match by propensity score (Section 7.5.A).

But despite these advantages, I recommend that you include all those variables that are associated with treatment assignment (option #1). The reason is that limiting the variables to those associated with outcome (option #2) or to true confounders (option #3) requires assessing the association between the variables and the outcome. This undercuts one of the advantages of propensity scores: that they can be calculated without regard to the outcome.[5]

As long as you do not consider how the variables that compose the propensity score (or the score itself) are related to outcome you can calculate the propensity score as many times as necessary without biasing your results. For example, a standard test for how well a propensity score works is to see whether cases and controls with similar propensity scores are similar on important covariates.

If you discover that there are differences between cases and controls with similar propensity scores on important covariates, you can recalculate the propensity score, perhaps including other variables, or a transformation (e.g., logarithmic transformation) of an existing variable, or an interaction between two variables to achieve better balance. Since these calculations are performed without consideration of the outcome, there is no risk of biasing your results by choosing the combination of variables for the propensity score that maximizes the difference between the groups on outcome.

Also, by including all those variables associated with treatment assignment, you do not risk missing a confounder. Missing a confounder is a much more

> Include in your propensity score all those variables that are associated with treatment group.

---

[4] Austin, P. C., Grootendorst, P., and Anderson, G. M. "A comparison of the ability of different propensity score models to balance measured variables between treated and untreated subjects: A Monte Carlo study." *Statist. Med.* **26** (2007): 734–53.

[5] Rubin, D. B. "Estimating causal effects from large data sets using propensity scores." *Ann. Intern. Med.* **127** (1997): 757–63.

significant problem than including a variable that is associated with group membership but is not a confounder.[6]

7.4 How do you assess the adequacy of a propensity score?

Once you have calculated a propensity score using those baseline variables that differ between the groups, there are three important checks on the adequacy of the score:

1 ability of propensity score to differentiate those who received the intervention from those who did not (Section 7.4.A);
2 whether there is sufficient overlap between the two groups on the propensity score (Section 7.4.B); and
3 whether the propensity score creates groups comparable on baseline characteristics (Section 7.4.C).

7.4.A Does the propensity score differentiate those who received the intervention from those who did not?

> **TIP**
>
> Use the c index to assess how well the propensity score differentiates those who received the intervention from those who did not.

To assess how well the propensity score differentiates those who receive the intervention from those who do not use the c index.[7] A value of 0.5 indicates that the model does not distinguish any better than chance. The maximum value is one. The higher the c index the better the model is at distinguishing the two groups. The c index is equal to the area under the receiver operating characteristics curve (ROC). A ROC curve can be constructed by plotting the sensitivity of the propensity score (in predicting who received the intervention) on the y-axis and (1–specificity) on the x-axis.

7.4.B Is there sufficient overlap between the two groups on the propensity score?

> There must be sufficient overlap of propensity score by treatment groups.

Although we want the propensity score to differentiate the two groups, for it to successfully adjust for baseline differences between the groups there also must be sufficient overlap of the propensity scores. One good way to assess this is to draw a box plot. For example, Landrum and Ayanian evaluated whether

---

[6] In some circumstances Austin *et al.* (footnote 4 in this chapter) found that reduction in bias was marginally greater when only true confounders were included in the propensity score than when including all variables associated with treatment selection. However, in other circumstances there was no difference. Overall, I think the dangers of biasing your propensity score by choosing variables based on their relationship with the outcome outweigh the potential advantages of including only true confounders.

[7] For how the c index is calculated see Katz, M. H. *Multivariable Analysis: A Practical Guide for Clinicians* (2nd edition). Cambridge: Cambridge University Press, 2006: p. 124.

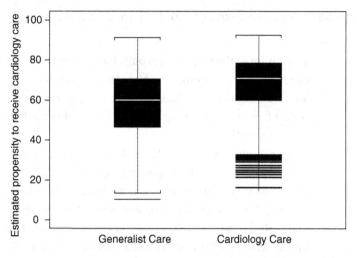

Figure 7.1

Comparison of box plots of propensity scores for likelihood of receiving cardiology care. Reprinted from Landrum, M.B. and Ayanian, J.Z. "Causal effect of ambulatory specialty care on mortality following myocardial infarction: A comparison of propensity score and instrumental variable analyses." *Health Serv. Outcomes Res. Methodol.* **2** (2001): 221–45, Figure 2, with kind permission from Springer Science and Business Media.

TIP

Assess overlap of propensity scores by using a box plot.

TIP

If comparison of groups by propensity scores shows many outliers recalculate the scores by including additional variables, transformations of existing variables, or interactions between variables.

---

specialty care decreased mortality among patients who suffered a myocardial infarction.[8] They calculated a propensity score, representing the probability of receiving care by a cardiologist, based on 41 clinical and provider characteristics.

As you can see in Figure 7.1, the propensity scores of patients who only received care by generalists were lower than the scores of those who received care by cardiologists – just as you would expect. But the scores overlapped. Also of interest, there were a larger number of outliers – patients who had a low predicted likelihood of seeing a cardiologist who nonetheless received cardiac specialty care. The outliers are shown with the straight lines outside the range of values demarcated with the brackets. This raises the possibility that other factors not included in the propensity score affected whether or not patients received care from a cardiac specialist. In such situations, try to recalculate the propensity scores by including additional variables, transformations of existing variables, or interactions between variables to achieve fewer outliers.

---

[8] Landrum, M. B. and Ayanian, J. Z. "Causal effect of ambulatory specialty care on mortality following myocardial infarction: A comparison of propensity score and instrumental variable analyses." *Health Serv. Outcomes Res. Methodol.* **2** (2001): 221–45.

7.4.C Does the propensity score create groups that are comparable on baseline characteristics?

In addition to the treatment groups having sufficient overlap on the propensity scores, the groups should also be balanced on important covariates within narrow strata of propensity scores. This can be assessed by stratifying subjects into at least five strata and comparing the values of subjects on important covariates by intervention group.

For example, in Section 4.3 I cited an observational study by Connors and colleagues assessing the impact of right heart catheterization (RHC) on mortality. The investigators found in bivariate results that patients who received an RHC had shorter survival compared to patients who did not receive an RHC (30-day survival was 62% versus 69%, respectively). However, patients who received right heart catheterization were also sicker at baseline so an unadjusted comparison between the two groups was not valid.

Therefore the authors calculated a propensity score from 65 baseline characteristics. To see whether the propensity score adjusted for important baseline differences between subjects receiving and not receiving an RHC, they divided the two groups into five strata (quintiles). As you can see in Figure 7.2, patients who received an RHC were similar on APACHE III scores (a composite measure of illness severity), blood pressure, and partial pressure of arterial oxygenation/fraction of inspired oxygen. The stratified comparison between the groups indicates the success of the propensity score in balancing baseline differences.

If the groups differ by propensity score on important covariates then you have two options. First, try to recalculate the propensity score by adding variables, transforming variables, or including interactions between variables, to achieve a propensity score on which the strata are more similar. Alternatively, include the covariates that are not sufficiently similar across treatment groups in the multivariable model in addition to the propensity score.

> **TIP**
>
> Stratify by propensity score using at least five strata to see whether subjects in different groups are similar on important covariates.

> **TIP**
>
> If baseline factors are not similar across strata recalculate the propensity score or include these covariates in the model predicting outcome.

7.5 How are propensity scores used to adjust for baseline differences?

Once a propensity score is created, there are four common ways to use it to adjust for baseline differences in the groups (Table 7.3).

These different methods are discussed below in Sections 7.5.A to 7.5.E.

7.5.A Matching cases using propensity scores

In the case of the study evaluating the effect of aspirin use on mortality (discussed above), the investigators used the propensity score as a matching

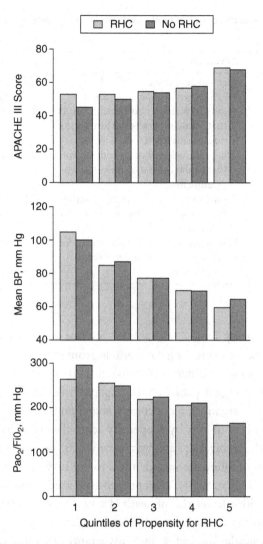

Figure 7.2   Patients receiving a right heart catheterization (RHC) and those who did not were stratified into five quintiles by propensity scores on APACHE III scores, blood pressure, and partial pressure of arterial oxygenation/fraction of inspired oxygen. Reproduced with permission from Connors, A.F., *et al.* "The effectiveness of right heart catheterization in the initial care of critically ill patients." *JAMA* **276** (1996): 889–97. Copyright © 1996 Amercian Medical Association. All rights reserved.

DEFINITION

Caliper is the maximum distance that can exist on a score between a case and a control and still consider them a match.

---

variable. Each aspirin user was matched to the non-aspirin user with the most similar propensity score. If no non-aspirin user could be identified whose propensity score was within 0.09 of the aspirin user's score, the aspirin user was excluded. The preset maximum difference that can exist between a case and a control for a match to be made is referred to as a caliper.

Table 7.3. Advantages and disadvantages of different methods of using propensity scores to adjust for baseline differences.

Methods of using propensity scores	Advantages	Disadvantages
Match cases and controls by propensity score	Best way to achieve comparable groups with propensity scores.	May decrease sample size and generalizability
Stratify cases and controls by propensity score	Allows inclusion of cases and controls that would otherwise be lost due to no close matches.	Residual bias.
Include the propensity score as an independent variable in multivariable model	Allows inclusion of cases and controls that would otherwise be lost due to no close matches.	Residual bias.
Use propensity scores to weight observations	Allows inclusion of cases and controls that would otherwise be lost due to no exact matches. May be less subject to misspecification of the regression models used to predict effect.	When propensity score is near zero or one, unrealistically extreme weights may be generated.

Comparing Table 7.4 to Table 7.2 you can see the success of matching by propensity score in creating comparable groups. Note that although there still are some significant differences between the two groups (e.g., men in the aspirin group had higher peak exercise capacity than men in the non-aspirin group) the groups are much more comparable than they were.

Matching subjects by propensity score dramatically changed the results of the study. In bivariate analysis, survival for persons who used aspirin during 3.1 years of follow-up was identical to the survival of persons who did not use aspirin (4.5% vs. 4.5%). With propensity-based matching, aspirin use was associated with a lower risk of death (4% vs. 8%, $P = 0.002$). This result is consistent with the results of randomized studies indicating that aspirin decreases cardiovascular morbidity. But, importantly, this study extends that finding to all-cause mortality and to patients seen in clinical practice (not just to those who would enter a clinical trial).

The method that Gum and colleagues used to match the cases (aspirin users) to the controls (non-aspirin users) – identifying for each case the control that had the closest propensity score – is the simplest way of matching cases and controls using propensity scores. However, in certain circumstances, it is critical to match the cases and controls not only on the propensity score but also on certain covariates. For example, it might be important to match cases and controls on sex.

For example, Stukel and colleagues assessed whether cardiac catheterization improved the survival of elderly patients following an acute myocardial

It is possible to match cases to controls on certain critical variables and then choose the control with the closest propensity score.

Table 7.4. Baseline characteristics of aspirin and non-aspirin users in propensity-matched pairs.

	Aspirin ($n = 1351$)	No aspirin ($n = 1351$)	P value
Demographics			
Age, mean (SD), yr	60 (11)	61 (11)	0.16
Men, no. (%)	951 (70)	974 (72)	0.33
Clinical history			
Diabetes, no. (%)	203 (15)	207 (15)	0.83
Hypertension, no. (%)	679 (50)	698 (52)	0.46
Tobacco use, no. (%)	161 (12)	162 (12)	0.95
Cardiac variables			
Prior coronary artery disease, no. (%)	652 (48)	659 (49)	0.79
Prior coronary artery bypass graft, no. (%)	251 (19)	235 (17)	0.42
Prior percutaneous coronary interv., no. (%)	166 (12)	147 (11)	0.25
Prior Q-wave MI, no. (%)	194 (14)	206 (15)	0.52
Atrial fibrillation, no. (%)	21 (2)	24 (2)	0.65
Congestive heart failure, no. (%)	79 (6)	89 (7)	0.43
Medication use			
Digoxin use, no. (%)	115 (9)	114 (9)	0.94
β-Blocker use, no. (%)	352 (26)	358 (26)	0.79
Diltiazem/verapamil use, no. (%)	223 (17)	223 (17)	0.99
Nifedipine use, no. (%)	127 (9)	144 (11)	0.28
Lipid-lowering therapy, no. (%)	281 (21)	271 (20)	0.63
ACE inhibitor use, no. (%)	209 (15)	214 (16)	0.79
Cardiovascular assessment and exercise capacity			
Body mass index, mean (SD), kg/m^2	29 (6)	29 (6)	0.83
Ejection fraction, mean (SD), %	51 (8)	51 (9)	0.65
Resting heart rate, mean (SD), beats/min	77 (13)	76 (14)	0.13
Systolic blood pressure, mean (SD), mmHg	141 (21)	141 (21)	0.68
Diastolic blood pressure, mean (SD), mmHg	85 (11)	86 (11)	0.57
Purpose of test to evaluate chest pain, no. (%)	153 (11)	159 (12)	0.72
Mayo Risk Index >1, no. (%)	1108 (82)	1110 (82)	0.92
Peak exercise capacity, mean (SD), METs			
Men	8.7 (2.5)	8.3 (2.5)	0.01
Women	6.5 (2.0)	6.7 (2.0)	0.13
Heart rate recovery, mean (SD), beats/min	28 (12)	28 (11)	0.82
Ischemic ECG charges with stress, no. (%)	231 (22)	223 (21)	0.64
Ejection fraction <40%, no. (%)	147 (11)	156 (12)	0.50
Stress-induced ischemia on echo, no. (%)	239 (18)	259 (19)	0.32
Fair or poor physical fitness, no. (%)	445 (33)	459 (34)	0.57

Data from: Gum, P.A., *et al.* "Aspirin use and all-cause mortality among patients being evaluated for known or suspected coronary artery disease: A propensity analysis." *JAMA* **286** (2001): 1187–94.

infarction.[9] The data were from a nonrandomized cohort of elderly persons. Following an analytic strategy similar to that of Gum and colleagues, they calculated a propensity score and then matched cases to controls whose

[9] Stukel, T. A., Fisher, E. S., Wennberg, D. E., Alter, D. A., Gottlieb, D. J., and Vermeulen, M. J. "Analysis of observational studies in the presence of treatment selection bias: Effects of invasive cardiac

propensity scores differed by less than 0.10 (caliper of 0.10). The one difference is that Stukel and colleagues required that cases and controls also were within 5 years of age of one another.

The major advantage of matching on propensity scores is that compared to other propensity score methods it generally provides the least biased estimates of treatment effect.[10]

> Matching by propensity score provides a better adjustment for baseline differences than other propensity score methods.

In the statistical world, advantages usually come with disadvantages. A disadvantage of matching by propensity score is that the matched sample may be smaller and not representative of the study population, thereby decreasing generalizability of results. Comparison of Table 7.2 and Table 7.4 demonstrates that the match resulted in keeping only 58% of the aspirin users (1351/2310) and 35% of the non-aspirin users (1351/3864). The implication is that, based on this study, we can only say that aspirin benefits people similar to those aspirin users whose propensity scores could be matched.

> Matching by propensity score may result in a smaller sample that is no longer representative of your study population.

7.5.B Stratifying analysis by propensity score

> To stratify by propensity score, group cases and controls with similar propensity scores into strata.

Since it is not always possible to find (near) exact matches on propensity score between cases and controls, you may instead stratify cases and controls by propensity scores. To use this method, create strata such that each stratum contains subjects with a similar propensity score.

Assuming that the subjects in each stratum have similar propensity scores and that all confounders were included in the calculation of the score then the subjects can be considered to have been randomly assigned to the study groups within each stratum. This is just a broadening of the concept that two subjects from different groups matched by propensity scores can be considered to have been randomly assigned to the group.

Once subjects are sorted into strata, the effectiveness of the intervention can be estimated for each stratum of patients. An overall measure of effectiveness can be estimated by averaging the within-stratum effects.

For example, Wang and colleagues compared mortality of elderly persons treated with conventional versus atypical antipsychotic medications.[11] As is true of the other nonrandomized studies in this section, there were sizable differences between the two groups; patients starting on conventional drugs

management on AMI survival using propensity score and instrument variable methods." *JAMA* **297** (2007): 278–85.

[10] Austin, P. C. "The performance of different propensity score methods for estimating marginal odds ratios." *Statist. Med.* **26** (2007): 3078–94.

[11] Wang, P. S., Schneeweiss, S., and Avorn, J. "Risk of death in elderly users of conventional vs. atypical antipsychotic medications." *N. Engl. J. Med.* **353** (2005): 2235–41.

were more likely to be male and non-white, and have congestive heart failure, ischemic heart disease other than myocardial infarction, and cancer than patients who were started on atypical antipsychotic medications.

To make the groups more comparable, the investigators calculated a propensity score for each patient and then used the propensity score to stratify their sample into deciles. In a proportional hazards model stratified by the deciles of the propensity score, mortality was greater at 180 days among users of conventional antipsychotics (hazard ratio = 1.37; 95% confidence interval 1.27–1.49) than among users of atypical antipsychotics.

A weakness of stratification is that you may have residual confounding. In other words, within each stratum of propensity score there may be important differences on baseline characteristics. To assess residual confounding, you can compare cases and controls on important baseline characteristics by strata.

> With stratification by propensity score there may be residual confounding.

In terms of how many strata to create, five strata have been shown to eliminate about 90% of the bias in unadjusted analyses.[12] An analysis comparing five strata to three or 10 equal-sized strata found similar results.[13]

> **TIP**
>
> Five strata eliminate 90% of the bias.

7.5.C Using propensity score as an independent variable in a multivariable model

Rather than using the propensity score to match cases or to create strata the score can be entered as an independent variable in a multivariable model. In other words, the propensity score would be an independent variable for which the value for each subject would be that subject's propensity score.

For example, Levy and colleagues assessed whether management by critical care physicians (intensivists) improved the mortality of intensive care unit (ICU) patients.[14] In unadjusted analysis, patients managed by intensivists had higher hospital mortality than patients not managed by intensivists (OR = 2.13; 95% CI 2.03–2.24; $P < 0.001$).

Intensivists reading this result will immediately protest that patients managed by intensivists tend to be sicker than those patients not managed by intensivists. Indeed, in this study, patients managed by intensivists were more likely to require ventilation in the first 24 hours of their ICU stay and were more likely to require continuous sedation than those not managed by intensivists.

[12] Rubin, D. B. "Estimating causal effects from large data sets using propensity scores." *Ann. Intern. Med.* **127** (1997): 757–63.

[13] Landrum, M. B. and Ayanian, J. Z. "Causal effect of ambulatory specialty care on mortality following myocardial infarction: A comparison of propensity score and instrumental variable analyses." *Health Serv. Outcomes Res. Methodol.* **2** (2001): 221–45.

[14] Levy, M. M., Rapoport, J., Lemeshow, S., Chalfin, D. B., Phillips, G., and Danis, M. "Association between critical care physician management and patient mortality in the intensive care unit." *Ann. Intern. Med.* **148** (2008): 801–9.

Also, ICUs that managed almost all their patients with intensivists were different (e.g., more likely to have an academic affiliation, sited in larger hospitals) than ICUs that managed few patients with intensivists. Often, academic hospitals receive the most challenging referrals; perhaps this accounts for why patients managed by intensivists have higher mortality. To adjust for these differences, the investigators calculated a propensity score based on 19 variables.

When the investigators entered the propensity score into a random-effects logistic model along with a scale measuring severity of illness, patients managed by intensivists still had higher hospital mortality (OR = 1.40; 95% CI 1.32–1.49; $P < 0.001$). So either there was residual confounding due to measured or unmeasured factors or there may be something about how intensivists treat patients (e.g., more procedures) that results in patients being more likely to die.

You may wonder why Levy and colleagues entered an adjustment for severity of illness in addition to the propensity score given that a number of variables related to severity of illness were included in the propensity score. The answer is that there still may be residual confounding and or misspecification even with the propensity variable in the model.

7.5.D Using the propensity score to weight observations

Another way to adjust for baseline differences is to use the propensity score to weight the multivariable analysis. For example, McNiel and colleagues used propensity-weighted multivariable analysis to assess the effectiveness of a mental health court.[15] As with the other nonrandomized studies discussed in this section, the challenge in assessing the effectiveness of the court was that those criminal defenders participating in the mental health court were different than those who received usual treatment. For example, those participating in the mental health court were more likely to be homeless and to have a severe mental disorder than those who received usual treatment.

To account for the differences between those participating in the court and those not participating, the investigators calculated a propensity score based on demographic characteristics, clinical variables, and criminal charges during the prior 12 months. The propensity score was then used to weight a proportional hazards model estimating the likelihood of recidivism; specifically (1) time to a new violent charge and (2) time to any new charge. The weight for a person receiving the intervention is the inverse of the propensity score; the weight for the control is the inverse of one minus the propensity score.

---

[15] McNiel, D. E. and Binder, R. L. "Effectiveness of a mental health court in reducing criminal recidivism and violence." *Am. J. Psychiatry* **64** (2007): 1395–403.

The investigators found that participation in the mental health court resulted in longer times without any charges for violent crimes or any new criminal charges.

Some analysts have found that using propensity scores to weight observations is less subject to misspecification of the regression models used to predict average causal effect than using propensity-based stratification.[16] A problem with weighting observations is that when the estimated propensity score is near zero or one, the weights may be extreme and unrealistic.[17]

7.5.E Choosing among the different methods of using propensity scores

> **TIP**
>
> Use matching by propensity score first and then consider stratifying by propensity score or including the propensity score as a covariate to improve generalizability.

> Different methods of using propensity scores should lead to similar results.

It is important to understand the advantages and disadvantages of the different approaches to using propensity scores. However, in practice, many people will use more than one method. Because matching produces the least biased estimates of treatment effect, there is a strong argument for using this method first. To overcome the limitation of decreased generalizability due to loss of subjects, researchers should also use the propensity scored to perform stratified analysis or include the propensity score as a covariate in a multivariable model.

In general, you should get similar results with different approaches. If you do, this will strengthen your findings. If the results differ, you will have learned something important about your data – perhaps that those cases for which matches are available are different from those cases that do not have appropriate matches.

7.6 What is instrumental variable analysis? How is it used to adjust for baseline differences between groups?

> Instrumental variable analysis offers the potential of adjusting for unknown or unmeasured confounders.

Instrumental variable analysis is a technique commonly used by economists to study the impact of social or economic policies (e.g., employment programs) on economic trends.[18] Its utility is that it can potentially mimic randomization by adjusting for **unknown** or **unmeasured** confounders. In contrast, multivariable analysis and propensity-score analysis can only adjust for **measured** confounders.

[16] Lunceford, J. K. and Davidian, M. "Stratification and weighting via the propensity score in estimation of causal treatment effects: A comparative study." *Statist. Med.* **23** (2004): 2937–60.

[17] Rubin, D. N. "Using propensity scores to help design observational studies: Application to the tobacco litigation." *Health Serv. Outcomes Res. Methodol.* **2** (2001): 169–88.

[18] Angrist, J. D., Imbens, G. W., and Rubin, D. B. "Identification of causal effects using instrumental variables." *J. Am. Stat. Assoc.* **91** (1996): 444–54; Newhouse, J. P. and McClellan, M. "Econometrics in outcomes research: The use of instrumental variables." *Annu. Rev. Public Health* **19** (1998): 17–34.

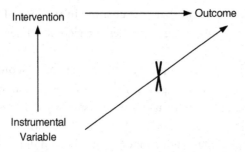

Figure 7.3   Relationship between an instrumental variable, an intervention, and an outcome.

The reason instrumental variable analysis has been used heavily in the economic arena is that economic policies are rarely randomized and economists are typically assessing the impact of these programs on the population. Recently, health researchers have noted the similarities between economic policy and health policy analysis, and shown increased interest in performing instrumental analysis to assess the impact of nonrandomized interventions.[19] For example, instrumental variable analysis can be used to assess the impact of health insurance (an intervention that is rarely randomized) on health outcomes.

DEFINITION

An instrumental variable is associated with the receipt of an intervention, but does not have any effect on the outcome except through its effect on whether or not the intervention is received.

An instrumental variable may simulate randomization.

To perform an instrumental variable analysis you must identify a variable that is associated with the receipt of an intervention, but does not have any effect on the outcome except through its effect on whether or not the intervention is received, as illustrated in Figure 7.3.

To illustrate how an instrumental variable can simulate randomization, let's look at a study of the effectiveness of mammography for women over the age of 70.[20] You might think that a question of this importance would have been addressed with a randomized study. Unfortunately the randomized controlled trials on this topic have generally excluded women over the age of 70 years.

---

[19] Sections 7.6–7.10 on instrumental analysis come with a warning: it is a non-intuitive technique. I have done my best to keep the explanation simple. Although it is important for certain nonrandomized designs most investigators have never used it, and perhaps you won't have cause to use it either. Try to read all the sections through rather than getting stuck on the details. For two general references on instrumental analysis see: Hernan, M. A. and Robins, J. M. "Instruments for causal inference: An epidemiologist's dream?" *Epidemiology* **17** (2006): 360–72; Greenland, S. "An introduction to instrumental variables for epidemiologists." *Int. J. Epidemiol.* **29** (2000): 722–9.

[20] Posner, M. A., Ash, A. S., Freund, K. M., Moskowitz, M. A., and Schwartz, M. "Comparing standard regression, propensity score matching, and instrumental variables for determining the influence of mammography on stage of diagnosis." *Health Serv. Outcomes Res. Methodol.* **2** (2001): 279–90.

Table 7.5. Does mammography result in earlier diagnosis of breast cancer?

	No mammogram	Mammogram
Early cancer	59%	81%
Late cancer	41%	19%
		$P = 0.001$

Data from Posner, M.A., *et al.* "Comparing standard regression, propensity score matching, and instrumental variables for determining the influence of mammography on stage of diagnosis." *Health Serv. Outcomes Res. Methodol.* **2** (2001): 279–90.

Table 7.6. Baseline differences between women with cancer by whether or not they received a mammogram.

	No mammogram	Mammogram	P value
Age at diagnosis	77	75	0.001
Charlson comorbidities			
Not hospitalized	27%	30%	
Hosp, no comorbidities	48%	54%	
At least one comorbidity	25%	16%	0.001
Race			
Black	6%	3%	
Non-black	94.8%	97%	0.001
Income (median of zip code)	$42 030	$41 137	0.061
Primary care visits	5	11	0.001

Data from Posner, M.A., *et al.* "Comparing standard regression, propensity score matching, and instrumental variables for determining the influence of mammography on stage of diagnosis." *Health Serv. Outcomes Res. Methodol.* **2** (2001): 279–90.

Therefore the investigators attempted to answer this question using an observational design. They matched Medicare records to a tumor registry to identify women who were diagnosed with breast cancer. They found that women who had mammography were more likely to present at an early stage of illness (Table 7.5). Does this prove that mammography is effective at detecting cancer earlier among older women?

If these data came from a study in which women had been randomized to mammography or not, it would be strong evidence that mammography resulted in earlier diagnosis of breast cancer. But this is an observational study. As you can see, in Table 7.6, there were substantial baseline differences between women who did and did not receive a mammogram.

To address these baseline differences, the investigators conducted an instrumental variable analysis. The instrumental variable was the region where the women lived. Women from Seattle were much more likely to have a mammogram (64%) than women who lived in Connecticut (50%) or in Atlanta (45%). Although it is known that there are substantial geographic differences in use of screening tests

Table 7.7. Estimation of the impact of mammography use on early diagnosis of breast cancer.

Variable	Multivariable model	Instrumental variable analysis
Age		
67–69 years	1.00 (reference)	1.00 (reference)
70–74 years	0.92 (0.75, 1.13)	0.92 (0.75, 1.13)
75–79 years	0.93 (0.75, 1.15)	0.93 (0.75, 1.16)
80–84 years	0.83 (0.66, 1.05)	0.82 (0.63, 1.07)
85+ years	1.02 (0.79, 1.32)	1.02 (0.70, 1.49)
Black	0.67 (0.50, 0.92)	0.70 (0.51, 0.98)
Comorbidities		
Not hospitalized	1.00 (reference)	1.00 (reference)
Hospital, no comorbidity	0.54 (0.45, 0.63)	0.55 (0.47, 0.65)
Hospital, comorbidity	0.48 (0.40, 0.59)	0.50 (0.40, 0.62)
High income	1.23 (1.08, 1.41)	1.22 (1.07, 1.41)
Region		
Connecticut	1.00 (reference)	–
Seattle	1.23 (1.06, 1.43)	–
Atlanta	1.17 (0.97, 1.41)	–
Primary care visits		
None	1.00 (reference)	1.00 (reference)
1–3	0.77 (0.62, 0.94)	0.76 (0.55, 1.04)
4–12	0.97 (0.80, 1.17)	0.95 (0.58, 1.58)
13+	0.79 (0.64, 0.98)	0.80 (0.45, 1.45)
Mammogram performed	2.97 (2.56, 3.45)	3.01 (1.09, 8.34)

Data from Posner, M. A., *et al.* "Comparing standard regression, propensity score matching, and instrumental variables for determining the influence of mammography on stage of diagnosis." *Health Serv. Outcomes Res. Methodol.* **2** (2001): 279–90.

there is no reason to believe that women are more likely to present at an early stage of cancer in one area than another due to factors other than screening test use.

Using region as an instrumental variable, the investigators found that receipt of mammography was associated with increased likelihood of being diagnosed with an early stage cancer. The results of the instrumental variable analyses are shown in Table 7.7 in the right column and the results of a simpler multivariable model are shown in the left.

As the odds ratio for the impact of mammography on early diagnosis is similar in the simple multivariable model (2.97) and the instrumental model (3.01), you may wonder what value the instrumental variable adds. The answer is that by using region to simulate randomization, we are simulating adjustment for unmeasured characteristics. The standard multivariable model only adjusts for those measured characteristics you see in Table 7.7. The fact that the point estimates are similar for the two analyses tells us that the relationship between mammography and early diagnosis does not appear to be biased by unmeasured confounders.

Table 7.8. Assumptions underlying instrumental analysis.

Assumption	How to assess
Instrumental variable is not associated with outcome except through its relationship with the intervention.	Cannot be tested directly and must be assumed based on theoretical considerations.
Instrumental variable is strongly associated with group assignment.	Perform multivariable analysis with receipt of intervention as dependent variable and instrumental variable along with other important baseline characteristics as the independent variables; repeat the analysis removing instrumental variable; compare the models.
Instrumental variable is not associated with baseline characteristics that are associated with outcome.	Assess the association between the instrumental variable and baseline characteristics known to be associated with outcome.
Instrumental variable has a monotonic relationship with intervention status: i.e., everyone who would get the intervention with a low score predicting intervention would also get the intervention with a high score predicting intervention.	Cannot be tested directly. Must be assumed based on theoretical considerations.

In the next section I will review the underlying assumptions of instrumental variable analysis, and then move on to how to conduct an instrumental variable analysis.

7.7 What are the underlying assumptions of instrumental variable analysis?

To conduct an instrumental variable analysis you need to identify an instrumental variable that fulfills four assumptions. Table 7.8 lists the four assumptions along with how to assess each of them. Greater detail is provided in the next four subsections.

7.7.A Is the instrumental variable unassociated with outcome except through its relationship with the intervention?

> Whether an instrumental variable is associated with outcome only through its relationship with group assignment cannot be tested directly.

It is impossible to prove that an instrumental variable is associated with an outcome variable only through its relationship with the intervention. Instead we choose instrumental variables that we believe, based on theoretical considerations, would be unlikely to be directly associated with the outcome.

To give you ideas for possible instrumental variables I have listed instrumental variables that have been used successfully in other studies along with the treatment assignments that they were used to predict and the outcome variable of the study (Table 7.9). The first one on the list is from the study of the effectiveness of mammography for older women discussed in Section 7.6. Note that

Table 7.9. Examples of instrumental variables used to estimate relationship between intervention and outcome.

Instrumental variable	Intervention	Outcome
Region where patient lives[a]	Mammogram	Stage of diagnosis
Rate of procedure (catheterization) in region where patient lives[b]	Cardiac catheterization	Mortality
Density of specialists (cardiologists) where patient lives[c]	Ambulatory cardiology care	Mortality
Physician preference[d]	Use of aprotinin during coronary artery bypass grafting	Mortality
Differential distance between specialty hospital (capable of performing catheterization) and nearest hospital in relation to patient's home[e]	Cardiac catheterization	Mortality
State unionization rate, state unemployment rate, and state tax rate (three instrumental variables) where patient lives[f]	Insurance	Health index
Generosity of Medicaid and AIDS Drug Assistance Program benefits in the state where the patient lives (six variables)[g]	Insurance	Mortality

[a] Posner, M. A., Ash, A. S., Freund, K. M., Moskowitz, M. A., and Schwartz, M. "Comparing standard regression, propensity score matching, and instrumental variables for determining the influence of mammography on stage of diagnosis." *Health Serv.Outcomes Res. Methodol.* **2** (2001): 279–90.

[b] Stukel, T. A., Fisher, E. S., Wennberg, D. E., Alter, D. A., Gottlieb, D. J., and Vermeulen, M. J. "Analysis of observational studies in the presence of treatment selection bias: Effects of invasive cardiac management on AMI survival using propensity score and instrumental variable methods." *JAMA* **297** (2007): 278–85.

[c] Landrum, M. B. and Ayanian, J. Z. "Causal effect of ambulatory specialty care on mortality following myocardial infarction: A comparison of propensity score and instrumental variable analyses." *Health Serv. Outcomes Res. Methodol.* **2** (2001): 221–45.

[d] Schneeweiss, S., Seeger, J. D., Landon, J., and Walker, A. M. "Aprotinin during coronary-artery bypass grafting and risk of death." *N. Engl. J. Med.* **358** (2008): 771–83.

[e] McCellan, M., McNeil, B. J., Newhouse, J. P. "Does more intensive treatment of acute myocardial infarction in the elderly reduce mortality: Analysis using instrumental variables." *JAMA* **272** (1994): 859–66.

[f] Goldman, D. P., Bhattacharya, J., McCaffrey, D. F., *et al.* "Effect of insurance on mortality in an HIV-positive population in care." *J. Am. Stat. Assoc.* **96** (2001): 883–94.

what the instrumental variables listed in Table 7.9 have in common (region, frequency of procedure use, density of specialists, physician preference, or state benefits) is that you wouldn't expect that these variables would influence health outcomes in ways other than affecting whether certain interventions occurred.

Note that several of these instrumental variables are sufficiently broad that they could be used for a range of outcomes. For example, distance to a specialty hospital, density of specialists in a particular area, or physician preferences are potential instrumental variables for a number of health service outcomes because a patient's location shouldn't affect health outcomes. Similarly, regional economic conditions may work as instrumental variables for health services research because the use of many procedures differs by region and not necessarily because of the characteristics of the patients within the region.

Although it is not possible to prove that an instrumental variable is associated with an outcome only through its relationship with the intervention, it is possible to test for violations of this assumption. Specifically, if an instrumental variable is associated with a factor that may influence treatment choices and affect the outcome, then the assumption is violated. For example, if a potential instrumental variable, community of residence, is associated with health status (perhaps certain communities attract a higher percentage of healthy people because of being near to athletic facilities), and health status influences whether a person receives an intervention as well as their mortality, then the community a patent lives in cannot be used as an instrumental variable.[21] (This issue is closely related to the assumption discussed in Section 7.7.C).

7.7.B Is the instrumental variable strongly associated with group assignment?

The stronger the association between an instrumental variable and receipt of the intervention, the more likely it is to work. The reason is that the stronger the instrumental variable, the larger is the group for whom the instrumental variable determines the treatment assignment and the more precise the treatment estimate will be.

> The stronger the association between an instrumental variable and receipt of the intervention the better.

The strength of the association between the instrumental variable and the group assignment is assessed by first performing a multivariable analysis with treatment assignment as the dependent variable (e.g., mammography would be the assignment variable in the study discussed in Section 7.6) and the instrumental variable (e.g., region), as well as potential confounders (e.g., age, comorbidities) as independent variables. Next, repeat the analysis removing the instrument from the model. Finally compare the two models (the one that includes the instrumental variable and the one that excludes the instrumental variable). If the treatment assignment is dichotomous (e.g., mammogram received or not), you might perform logistic regression. If the treatment assignment is interval (e.g., number of visits), you might perform multiple linear regression.

> Stronger instrumental variables result in more precise treatment estimates.

> Compare a model with the instrumental variable to a model without the instrumental variable; the chi-squared value divided by the degrees of freedom should be at least 20 or the *F* value should be at least 10.

As a rule of thumb, the chi-squared value divided by the degrees of freedom for the comparison of the logistic models with and without the instrumental variable should be at least 20. Alternatively, the F values for a linear regression model with and without the instrumental variable should be at least 10.[22]

In the analysis of the impact of mammography on stage of breast cancer diagnosis, the chi-squared statistic was 53.0 with two degrees of freedom. This

[21] Newhouse, J. P. and McClellan, M. "Econometrics in outcomes research: The use of instrumental variables." *Annu. Rev. Public Health* **19** (1998): 17–34.

[22] Staiger, D. and Stock, J. H. "Instrumental variables regression with weak instruments." Econometrica **63** (1997): 557–86; Posner, M. A., Ash, A. S., Freund, K. M., Moskowitz, M. A., and Schwartz, M. "Comparing standard regression, propensity score matching, and instrumental variables for

exceeds our threshold of 20 for the quotient of the chi-square divided by the degrees of freedom.

7.7.C Is the instrumental variable associated with baseline characteristics that are associated with the outcome?

For an instrumental variable analysis to be valid there should be no association between the instrumental variable and baseline characteristics associated with the outcome. To understand why, remember that our goal with instrumental variable analysis is to simulate a randomized study.

> There should be no association between the instrumental variable and baseline characteristics associated with the outcome.

One of the major advantages of randomization is that it tends to produce groups that are comparable with respect to baseline characteristics (Section 4.2). The same should be true of an instrumental variable.

To test the association between the instrumental variable and the baseline characteristics associated with outcome, perform a bivariate analysis. If your instrumental variable is dichotomous or categorical (e.g., region in the mammography study), you can simply compare across categories. If it is continuous, you will need to divide the samply into categories to determine whether the instrumental variable is associated with prognostically important baseline characteristics.

For example, in Section 7.5.A, I described a study by Stukel and colleagues that used propensity scores to evaluate the efficacy of cardiac catheterization in patients who had previously suffered a myocardial infarction (heart attack). They also used instrumental variable analysis to answer the same question. Their instrumental variable was regional catheterization rate. The rate of cardiac catheterization following a myocardial infarction varied widely (29% to 82.3%) across the United States. For regional catheterization rate to function as an instrumental variable, prognostically important variables should be similar across regions.

To test whether this were true of their data, the investigators divided their sample into five groups of approximately equal numbers of patients (Table 7.10). The proportion of patients in each group receiving catheterization (ranging from 42.8% in the first quintile to 65.0% in the fifth quintile) closely correlated with the regional catheterization rate, indicating that regional catheterization rate was strongly associated with whether an individual patient received catheterization. If you compare the patients in the five groups you can see that their baseline characteristics are similar (although not identical).

If the instrumental variable is associated with variables that are prognostically related to the outcome, you may still proceed with the analysis. However, you will need to adjust for these variables in the model. This is

determining the influence of mammography on stage of diagnosis." *Health Serv. Outcomes Res. Methodol.* **2** (2001): 279–90.

Table 7.10. Baseline characteristics across quintiles of regional cardiac catheterization rate.

	Quintile (range) of regional cardiac catheterization rate, %				
	1 (29.2–48.1)	2 (48.2–53.0)	3 (53.1–56.3)	4 (56.4–60.2)	5 (60.3–82.3)
No. of patients	24 872	24 184	24 718	24 063	24 287
Cardiac catheterization rate	42.8	50.6	54.7	58.0	65.0
Acute myocardial infarction severity	26.1	26.0	25.5	25.3	24.6
Demographics					
Age range, yr					
65–74	53.3	54.4	54.6	55.6	55.6
75–84	46.7	45.6	45.4	44.4	44.4
Men	53.7	54.2	55.0	55.6	56.4
Black	4.1	8.1	6.3	5.5	5.4
Social Security income > $2600	30.4	28.2	33.4	27.9	29.1
Comorbidities					
History of angina	50.1	48.3	47.8	47.6	44.0
Previous myocardial infarction	30.1	29.8	29.2	28.7	26.9
Previous revascularization	16.5	18.6	20.8	20.2	22.1
Congestive heart failure	18.4	18.0	17.3	16.9	15.1
Diabetes mellitus	32.9	32.5	32.3	31.3	30.0
Peripheral vascular disease	10.5	10.9	11.0	10.4	10.0
Chronic obstructive pulmonary disease	21.1	20.2	20.3	20.3	20.7
Smoker	16.7	16.7	17.0	18.0	17.9
AMI clinical presentation characteristics					
Non-ST-segment elevation AMI	40.4	41.2	40.5	39.3	39.0
Shock	1.6	1.6	1.6	1.7	1.7
Hypotension	2.8	2.9	2.6	2.8	2.7
Received CPR	1.6	1.7	1.7	1.8	1.7
Peak creatinine kinase >1000 U/L	30.3	30.5	30.4	31.7	32.6

Data from Stukel, T.A., *et al.* "Analysis of observational studies in the presence of treatment selection bias: Effects of invasive cardiac management on AMI survival using propensity score and instrumental variable methods." *JAMA* **297** (2007): 278–85.

the same approach that would be necessary if you performed a randomized controlled trial, and by chance there were important baseline differences.

The problem with this approach is that if you have strong differences in prognostic characteristics it raises the question of whether the instrumental variable is effectively simulating randomization. Continuing with the analogy to randomization, although you can by bad luck obtain unequal groups, if there were strong differences between the groups you would wonder whether there were a problem with your randomization.

You may find that an instrumental variable is associated with baseline differences but that these differences are not associated with the outcome. For example, if the instrumental variable was density of specialists and the outcome were mortality, the density of specialists may be associated with urbanicity of

TIP

It is not a problem if the instrumental variable is associated with baseline differences that are not associated with the outcome.

the area. Presumably, urbanicity is not associated with mortality. Therefore, this should not pose a problem for an instrumental variable analysis.

7.7.D Instrumental variable has a monotonic relationship with intervention status

This assumption sounds much more complicated than it is. What it means is that persons who would get the intervention with a given score predicting intervention would also get the intervention with a higher score predicting intervention.[23] In other words, having a higher score on the prediction would not work against the person obtaining the intervention. This assumption cannot be tested but has to be assumed on theoretical grounds to be true.

7.8 How is instrumental variable analysis performed?

The first job in conducting an instrumental variable analysis is to prove that the instrumental variable fits the two assumptions that can be empirically tested for: strength of association between the instrumental variable and the group assignment (Section 7.7.B) and lack of association between the instrumental variable and baseline characteristics associated with outcome (Section 7.7.C). For the two that cannot be proven, consider whether the instrument variable fits the assumption on theoretical grounds.

Having convinced yourself that the instrument fulfills the four assumptions, you can perform the analysis. As is true of propensity models, instrumental variable analysis involves two stages. In stage one the instrumental variable, along with any other predictors of the intervention, is used to predict the likelihood of receiving the intervention for each subject. In stage two, these predicted values replace the actual intervention assignment for each subject and are used to estimate the impact of the intervention on the outcome.

Look back at Table 7.7. Note that the confidence intervals for the estimates of the impact of mammogram use on breast cancer diagnosis were much wider for the model using the instrumental variable than for the multivariable model. Because instrumental variable analysis replaces the actual treatment assignment of each subject with the prediction of treatment assignment based on the first-stage model, the estimates tend to be less precise (have larger standard errors).[24]

Note also that in the instrumental variable model the instrumental variable is not entered into the model. The reason is that the instruments are assumed

---

[23] Angrist, J. D., Imbens, G. W., and Rubin, D. B. "Identification of causal effects using instrumental variables." *J. Am. Stat. Assoc.* **91** (1996): 444–54.

[24] Fortney, J. C., Steffick, D. E., Burgess, J. F., Maciejewski, M. L., and Petersen, L. A. "Are primary care services a substitute or complement for specialty and inpatient services?" *Health Serv. Res.* **40** (2005): 1422–42.

to be unrelated to outcome except through their effect on outcome; therefore, it is not necessary to adjust the model for them.

7.9 What are the limitations of instrumental variable analysis?

The marginal population is the proportion of subjects who received the intervention based on their value on the instrumental variable.

Instrumental variable analysis can only be used to analyze the impact of an intervention on a population, not on individuals.

LATE is the average survival benefit for having the intervention among persons for whom the instrument determined that they received the intervention.

Certainly, the biggest limitation to instrumental variable analysis is identifying instrumental variables that fit the assumptions listed in Table 7.8.

Beyond this, the results of an instrumental variable only apply to those patients whose treatment status is determined by their value on the instrumental variable.[25] This is called the **marginal** population.

In the case of the study of mammography, the benefit is demonstrated only for the population of women whose receipt of mammography is influenced by living in an area where mammography is commonly provided. The results do not pertain to women who would never receive mammography or who would always receive mammography no matter where they lived. For these reasons, instrumental variable analysis cannot be used to predict the impact of interventions on specific individuals.

In the case of a study where you are predicting survival differences, the survival difference for the marginal population is referred to as the local average treatment effect (LATE).[26] It is the average benefit gained by having the intervention among persons for whom the instrument determined that they received the intervention. For example, the study of the impact of cardiac catheterization on mortality (Section 7.5.A) found that cardiac catheterization was associated with a 16% decrease in mortality (adjusted RR 0.84; 95% CI 0.79–0.90). This is the average effect of cardiac catheterization for those persons for whom regional catheterization rate determined their receipt of catheterization.

Given this similarity, how well do instrumental variables simulate randomization? The answer depends on how sure you are that the instrumental variable does not have any effect on the outcome except through its effect on the intervention. When you randomize, assuming you have done so without bias, you can have great confidence that the randomization process is not associated with the outcome. In fact, the outcome is not known at the time of the randomization process. This is not the case with instrumental variable analysis, which is performed using retrospective data and the outcome is known.

Moreover, since an instrumental variable is not randomly assigned, you cannot take it on faith that there is no relationship between the instrumental

---

[25] Harris, K. M. and Remler, D. K. "Who is the marginal patient? Understanding instrumental variables estimates of treatment effects." *Health Serv. Res.* **33** (1998): 1337–60.

[26] Imbens, G. W. and Angrist, J. D. "Identification and estimation of local average treatment effects." *Econometrica* **62** (1994): 467–75.

variable and the outcome other than through group assignment. Worse yet, you cannot assess whether the instrumental variable is unrelated to outcome except through its relationship to the outcome. Nonetheless, because instrumental variable analysis is the only method available for adjusting observational data for unmeasured characteristics, it is an important tool.

7.10 How do the results of multivariable adjustment alone, propensity scores, and instrumental variable analysis compare?

Several studies have compared the results of analyses using multivariable analysis alone, multivariable analysis with propensity scores, and instrumental variable analysis. For example, the study of the impact of mammography on stage of cancer diagnosis discussed in Section 7.6 used both propensity analysis and instrumental variable analysis; the two techniques produced similar results.

In contrast, the study of the impact of cardiac catheterization on mortality described in Section 7.7.C found that standard multivariable analysis and propensity-based matched analysis indicated a much stronger effect of cardiac catheterization than an instrumental variable analysis. The investigators interpreted this difference as being due to instrumental variable analysis being less biased. However, not all experts agree.[27]

My own view is that there is too little experience to conclude that instrumental variable analysis is less biased than these other methods, although I think it is a promising technique for addressing problems that cannot be addressed with these other methods.

My general advice is when possible analyze your data using more than one method. When different methods produce similar answers you can have greater faith in the answer. When they produce different answers, focus on why they produced different answers rather than which method is better.

> When different methods produce different answers, focus on why, rather than which method is better.

Also, remember that instrumental variable analysis, and to a lesser extent propensity analysis, are conceptually difficult procedures. Many readers will have difficulty understanding them. For this reason if your intervention can be evaluated adequately with multivariable analysis alone there may be no reason to perform a more complicated analysis.

7.11 What is sensitivity analysis?

> The point of sensitivity analysis is to see how the results change with varying the inputs.

Sensitivity analysis refers to a broad group of analyses in which the investigator varies certain inputs to see how such changes affect the results.

---

[27] D'Agostino, R. B. Jr. and D'Agostino, R.B. Sr. "Estimating treatment effects using observational data." *JAMA* **297** (2007): 314–16; D'Agostino, R. B. Jr. and D'Agostino, R. B. Sr. "Using observational data to estimate treatment effects – Reply." *JAMA* **297** (2007): 2079.

In the context of this chapter, we are interested in a particular type of sensitivity analysis: how strong and how prevalent would an unmeasured confounder have to be to change the conclusion of the study?

If, for example, we assume that there is an unmeasured confounder present among 20% of your subjects that is correlated with the intervention you are studying at 0.30, how strong would its relationship to outcome have to be to change your results? If the answer is not very strong, than your results may be biased by an unmeasured confounder because it is easy to miss weak confounders. If the answer is that the unmeasured confounder has to be very strong, then it is much less likely that such a confounder exists and yet investigators in the field are unaware of it.

For example, colleagues of mine and I at the San Francisco Department of Health conducted an observational study to evaluate the impact of housing on mortality of homeless persons with AIDS by matching a supportive housing registry to an AIDS registry.[28] We identified 70 homeless persons who received supportive housing after an AIDS diagnosis and 606 homeless persons who were not housed by the program. To determine whether receipt of housing was associated with decreased mortality, we performed a proportional hazards model adjusting for age, ethnicity, CD4 count at time of diagnosis, and HIV risk group. We found that mortality was reduced by 80% for persons who received supportive housing (RH = 0.20; 95% confidence intervals 0.05 to 0.81).

Although we adjusted for a number of potential confounders, the question remained whether there could be some unmeasured confounder that explained why persons who received supportive housing were less likely to die. We had no good candidates for an instrumental variable analysis. Instead, we performed a sensitivity analysis. We found that an unmeasured confounder would need to exist at a prevalence level of 70%, be correlated at 0.5 with not receiving supportive housing, and predict at least a nine-fold increase in risk to eliminate the beneficial impact of supportive housing on mortality. Although not impossible, it is unlikely that such a strong and prevalent confounder exists and yet we (and other investigators in our field) are not aware of it. Other prevalence levels and correlations with receipt of supportive housing were even less plausible.[29]

> It is easy to miss weak confounders.

---

[28] Schwarcz, S. K., Hsu, L. C., Vittinghoff, E., Vu, A., Bamberger, J. D., and Katz, M. H. "Impact of housing on the survival of persons with AIDS." *BMC Public Health* **9** (2009): 220.

[29] Our manuscript provides a formula in the appendix for calculating how different combinations of prevalence of risk factor and correlation with the risk factor would result in different strengths of a confounder necessary to eliminate the effect of an intervention on an outcome. Based on these scenarios, you can determine how plausible it would be for a confounder to explain your results.

Time series analysis

8.1 How do I use time series analysis to analyze how an intervention affects a series of observations over time?

For some interventions, the best way of determining whether they are effective is to observe whether they cause a change in the pattern of a series of observations over time. For example, you may want to know whether an intervention affects the number of births, the number of deaths, the number of infections, or the number of accidents during a three-year period in a particular city. Methods for examining trends in a series of observations are called time series analyses. The specific method for determining whether an intervention affects a series of observations is called interrupted time series analysis.[1]

Although the name "interrupted time series analysis" sounds complicated this method is just a fancy pre-intervention versus post-intervention design (Section 1.2.A) with a lot of pre-intervention and post-intervention points; the "interruption" is the intervention. The idea is that with a series of measurements over time you can detect changes in pattern. When a change coincides with the start of an intervention, it suggests that the intervention has had an effect.

Interrupted time series analyses are used most commonly to evaluate non-randomized interventions. Often the outcome data come from an administrative dataset (e.g., registries of birth, death, accidents). However, the method can be used for randomized designs as well.

To perform time series analyses the data must be in the form of events per time and the intervals must be equally spaced (e.g., births per day, accidents per week, infections per month). The data can be a series of observations of a population (e.g., births per month in a particular country) or a single person (e.g., number of times per day that a person experiences an episode of pain).

[1] For a good introduction to interrupted time series, see: Shadish, W. R., Cook, T. D., and Campbell, D. T. *Experimental and Quasi-experimental Designs for Generalized Causal Inference.* Boston: Houghton Mifflin, 2002: pp. 171–206.

Time series data may be a count, a mean value, or a proportion per time interval.

Besides count data other kinds of data that can be used with time series are mean value (e.g., mean number of prescriptions dispensed per subject) or proportion (e.g., proportion of subjects who received HIV risk-reduction counseling), so long as the outcomes can be measured on a time scale (e.g., mean number of prescriptions dispensed per patient per month; proportion of subjects receiving counseling per year).

To increase the likelihood that the changes that appear to be temporally related to the intervention are actually related to the intervention, it is helpful to have a series of observations over the same period of time in a setting where the intervention did not occur. With a comparison group, an interrupted time series analysis is a fancy pre-intervention versus post-intervention with concurrent controls (Section 1.2.B).

Segmental regression analysis is used to determine whether the changes in a time series at the point of interruption (the intervention) are greater than would be expected by chance.

With or without controls, it is desirable to test whether the changes that occur following an intervention are greater than would be expected by chance. The analytic tool for determining whether the change is greater than would be expected by chance is called segmental regression analysis.

To better understand the concepts of time series, interrupted time series, segmental regression analysis, and the use of control groups, let's examine an evaluation of a change in HIV testing policy in San Francisco.[2] Prior to May 2006 the San Francisco Public Health Department required written patient consent for HIV testing in its medical settings; beginning in May 2006 only verbal agreement was required. The new policy was instituted because we believed that written consent (as opposed to verbal agreement) was a barrier to persons receiving testing. The change in policy applied only to public health facilities in San Francisco and not to other providers in the county.

Figure 8.1 shows a graphic presentation of time series data. Each dot represents the number of HIV tests per patient visits at public health settings. The vertical line represents the interruption of the series in May 2006 when the new policy went into effect.

Visually inspecting the time series it would appear that in the period July 2004 to May 2006 the number of tests performed was gradually increasing, but that at the interruption – May 2006 when the new policy began – there was an increase in the number of tests performed, and an acceleration in the rate of increase.

This point is made in Figure 8.2, which is the same data as Figure 8.1, except I have added two segmental regression lines. The lines help you to see the sharp

---

[2] Zetola, N. M., Grijalva, C. G., Gertler, S., *et al.* "Simplifying consent for HIV testing is associated with an increase in HIV testing and case detection in highest risk groups, San Francisco January 2003–2007." *PloS One* **3** (2008): e2591. Some of the analyses reported here were not in the published article, but were supplied by the lead author.

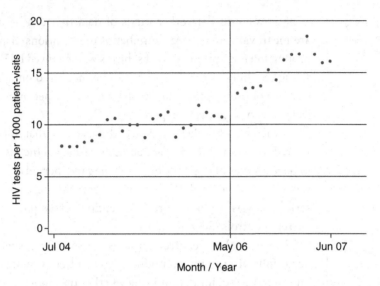

Figure 8.1   Number of HIV tests performed per month at San Francisco public health facilities; the change in HIV testing policy occurred in May 2006.

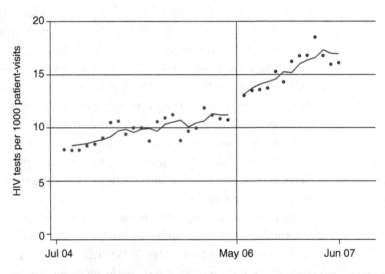

Figure 8.2   Number of HIV tests performed per month at San Francisco public health facilities with segmental regression lines.

increase in the level of testing following the change of policy in May 2006. The steeper slope of the top line compared to the bottom line illustrates how testing increased more rapidly following the policy change than it had prior to the change.

Each segment of a
segmental regression
analysis can be defined
in terms of level and
slope.

The transition period or
lag time is the period
between the initiation
of the intervention
and the time the
intervention would be
expected to take hold.

Segmental regression
analysis can adjust
for factors other than
the intervention that
could have caused
changes in the series of
observations.

Time series models
can adjust for
the correlation
between sequential
observations.

Note that each of the two segments seen on Figure 8.2 can be defined using two parameters: the level (where the segment starts) and the slope. To conduct an interrupted time series analysis we must also specify a transition period or lag time when no significant change is anticipated. The analysis of the new HIV testing policy assumed that the policy change took one month to become standard practice and therefore May of 2006 was considered the transition month and data from that month were excluded.

To statistically determine the impact of an intervention we use segmental regression analysis[3] to see whether the level and the slope changed after the intervention, compared to the segment prior to the intervention. In the case of the data shown in Figure 8.2, we found that both the level and the slope increased significantly after the intervention.

In addition to determining whether the level and slope have significantly changed after the intervention, segmental regression analysis can also be used to adjust for other factors that may have changed during the study period. For example, segmental regression analyses can adjust for seasonal changes (as long as you have data from more than one year!) or changes in the population (e.g., more homeless persons seeking care).

In the case of the analysis of the HIV testing policy change, we adjusted for age, race, language, gender, homelessness status, insurance, and health care setting. With these terms in the model, we found that the average monthly rate of HIV tests increased by 4.38 tests over what would have been predicted by the baseline trend ($P < 0.001$).

An important aspect of time series data is that the error terms associated with each observation are not independent. Indeed, error terms of sequential observations are likely to be correlated. Special methods are needed to incorporate this dependence, otherwise the standard errors will be underestimated and the statistical significance will be overestimated. The most commonly used model for analyzing time series data with correlated errors is autoregressive integrative moving average (ARIMA), which uses prior values to estimate later values. By correctly modeling the errors (or noise) we can determine the effectiveness of the intervention.[4]

[3] Segmental regression analysis is a difficult topic. An excellent introduction is: Wagner, A. K., Soumerai, S. B., Zhang, F., and Ross-Degnan, D. "Segmented regression analysis of interrupted time series studies in medication use research." *J. Clin. Pharm. Ther.* **27** (2000): 299–309.

[4] For more on ARIMA see: Hartmann, D. P., Gottman, J. M., Jones, R. R., *et al.* "Interrupted times-series analysis and its application to behavioral data." *J. Applied Behav. Anal.* **13** (1980): 543–59; Garson, C.D. *Time Series Analysis*, 2008. http://faculty.chass.ncsu.edu/garson/PA765/time.htm; Cochrane Effective Practice and Organisation of Care Group. "EPOC methods paper: Including interrupted time series (ITS) designs in a EPOC review." 1998. http://epoc.cochrane.org/Files/Website/Reviewer%20Resources/inttime.pdf.

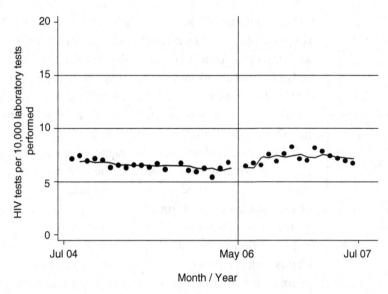

Figure 8.3   HIV tests at a San Francisco university-based medical center that did not change its HIV testing policy.

Despite the ability of segmental regression analysis to adjust for changes in the population over time and auto-correlation, the results of the HIV testing analysis still leave an important question. Could there be some other factor that occurred at the same time as the new HIV testing policy that truly accounted for the increase in testing rates other than the variables the investigators adjusted for? For example, could there be some other factor that was increasing HIV testing at all hospitals in San Francisco or could there be some other factor that was increasing all kinds of tests in the San Francisco public health system. To explore these possibilities the investigators used two controls: HIV testing at a university-based medical center that did not change its HIV testing policy (Figure 8.3) and hematocrit testing within the public health system (Figure 8.4). Segmental regression analysis showed no significant change following May 2006 in the rates of testing for these controls.

Although segmental regression analysis of interrupted time series data is a powerful tool, if you are using it to analyze data from a nonrandomized study, all the same limitations exist as with any analysis of observational data: you cannot exclude confounding due to some unmeasured factor. In the case of this study, we cannot completely exclude the possibility that the increase in HIV testing rates seen in the San Francisco public facilities but not in the university hospital was due to some other factor.

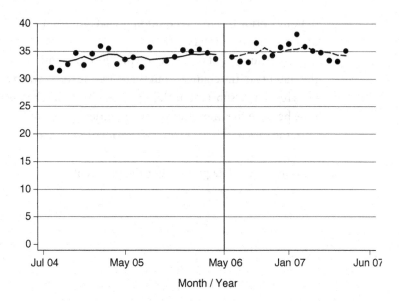

Figure 8.4   Hematocrit tests per month at San Francisco public health facilities.

Nonetheless, this study had a major impact. The data were cited as supporting evidence for a legislative bill to change HIV testing policy in California. The bill passed and was signed by the Governor. Beginning in 2008 in California HIV testing could be done as an opt-out test similar to other medical tests. In other words, a patient would be told by the physician of the intention to order HIV testing, and the patient could tell the doctor if he or she did not want the test.

8.2 How many observations are needed for performing an interrupted time series analysis?

TIP

For interrupted time series analysis you should have at least 20 data points prior to the interruption.

As with many statistical questions, the general answer is easy and the specific answer is hard. The general answer is the more data points you have the better. Classically, experts argued that you should have at least 100 data points.[5] However, many valid analyses have been published with fewer.

For a valid ARIMA model, there should be at least 20 data points prior to the interruption.[6] The reason for wording the guidance in terms of the number

---

[5] Shadish, W. R., Cook, T. D., and Campbell, D. T. *Experimental and Quasi-Experimental Designs for Generalized Causal Inference*. Boston: Houghton Mifflin, 2002: p. 174.

[6] Cochrane Effective Practice and Organisation of Care Group. "EPOC methods paper: Including interrupted time series (ITS) designs in a EPOC review." 1998. http://epoc.cochrane.org/Files/Website/Reviewer%20Resources/inttime.pdf; England, E. "How interrupted time series analysis can evaluate guideline implementation." *Pharm. J.* **275** (2005): 344–7; Hartmann, D. P., Gottman, J. M., Jones, R. R., *et al.* "Interrupted times-series analysis and its application to behavioral data." *J. Applied Behav. Anal.* **13** (1980): 543–59.

of points prior to the intervention is that you need a solid baseline to evaluate changes due to an intervention.

A large number of points following the intervention is useful for establishing the stability of the change – but there may be times when an intervention really does result in a substantial change in level, but the change is not sustained over time because the impact of the intervention dissipates.

In the case of the study on the impact of a change in HIV testing consent on number of tests ordered (Section 8.1), we had 22 data points before the intervention and 13 data points after the intervention.

Special topics

9.1 What methods are available for evaluating interventions that do not occur to all subjects at the same time?

It is common in observational cohorts to have different subjects start an intervention at different times, with some subjects never receiving it. This is particularly common when new medications are introduced into practice.

In situations such as these, you may have no subjects on the medication (prior to approval) and then a gradual uptake in medication use. Let's assume you want to evaluate the impact of a new medication designed to prevent osteoporosis. Your outcome is occurrence of a pathologic fracture (yes/no). How would you do it?

At first blush you might think that you could compare the number of fractures in the 280 persons who took the drug to the number of fractures among the 720 persons who did not take the drug.

But this would be wrong from several points of view. First, for those people who dropped out we would only know what happened to them prior to the drop-out (e.g., whether they started taking the medicine, that they didn't develop a fracture) . By year 5, some of them may have begun the medicine and some may have had a fracture. We could exclude dropouts from our analysis but then we would lose 15% of our total sample. And what about the deaths that occurred during the study prior to a fracture? Had these people lived some of them may have started taking the medicine and some of them may have had a fracture. Do we exclude the deaths as well and lose another 21% of our sample?

Survival bias occurs when an intervention appears to work because people who live longer are more likely to receive it.

To minimize the impact of losses to follow-up we could use survival analysis. This would allow us to censor subjects when they dropped out; in other words, we would maintain the benefit of the time they were under observation (Section 6.4.G). The problem with this solution is that it creates survival bias. Specifically, persons who survive longer have a higher chance of receiving the new medication (because, as you can see in Table 9.1, rates of medication use are increasing over time in the cohort). Therefore, people who received a new

Table 9.1. Uptake of a hypothetical medicine to prevent osteoporosis in a hypothetical cohort of 1000 patients.

	Year one	Year two	Year three	Year four	Year five
Cumulative subjects taking medicine	0	90	170	225	280
Cumulative pathologic fractures	10	15	25	35	40
Cumulative drop outs (before a fracture)	40	60	85	100	150
Cumulative deaths (before a fracture)	50	100	140	190	210
Fracture-free sample size at end of year	900	825	750	675	600

medication within the cohort will tend to do better even if the medication does not work, simply because they lived long enough to receive the medication.

To avoid survival bias in cohort studies, use time-dependent covariates to represent the different times at which subjects begin the intervention. With a time-dependent covariate, the variable changes value at the time that the intervention occurs. In the case of a new medication, every one in the cohort illustrated in Table 9.1 would have a value of zero at the start of the study and then the variable would switch to a value of 1 at the time the subject begins the medication. If the subject never begins the medication during the study the value remains zero for that subject throughout the study. It is also possible to construct time-dependent variables that change value back and forth (if, for example, a person starts and stops taking a medication).

For example, De Martino and colleagues used time-dependent covariates to evaluate the effectiveness of antiretroviral therapy for children with perinatal HIV-1 infection.[1] The investigators followed children born between 1980 and 1997; the outcome of the study was survival.

As you can see in Figure 9.1, the use of antiretroviral therapy increased over the study period. In the first panel you can see that none of the children was taking antiviral therapy in 1987 and over 80% were taking it by 1998. Moreover, during this period, therapy intensified. At first monotherapy grew in numbers, then double combination therapy, and in the later years triple combination therapy.

Had the investigators treated antiretroviral therapy as a yes/no variable, receipt of therapy would have certainly been associated with longer survival

> **TIP**
>
> Use time-dependent covariates to avoid survival bias in cohort studies.

> Time-dependent covariates change value during a study.

---

[1] De Martino, M., Tovo, P.-A., Balducci, M., *et al.* "Reduction in mortality with availability of antiretroviral therapy for children with perinatal HIV-1 infection." *JAMA* **284** (2000): 190–7.

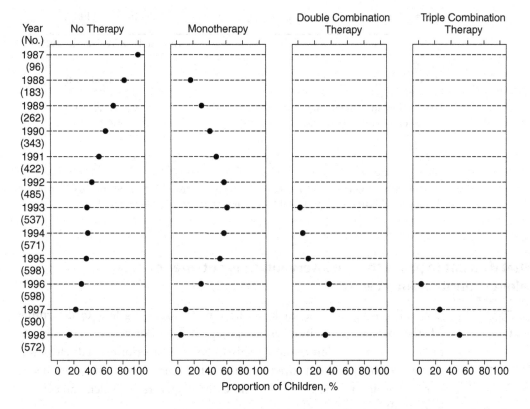

Figure 9.1

Proportion of children receiving antiretroviral treatment over time. Reproduced with permission from De Martino, M., *et al.* "Reduction in mortality with availability of antiretroviral therapy for children with perinatal HIV-1 infection." *JAMA* **284** (2000): 190–7. Copyright © 2000 American Medical Association. All rights reserved.

because children alive in the later years were more likely to receive treatment, especially triple combination therapy, which wasn't used prior to 1997 and is markedly more effective than other types of therapy.

Therefore, the investigators created three time-dependent variables: one for monotherapy, one for double combination therapy, and one for triple combination therapy; the value for each of the three variables was set to zero for each subject at the start of the study and became one at the time (if ever) the therapy was begun. The results are shown in Table 9.2.

Time-dependent covariates do not have to be dichotomous. Time-dependent variables can be interval measures such as systolic blood pressure or CD4 lymphocyte counts. At each point at which the variable is measured it takes on a different value.

Table 9.2. Effect of antiretroviral therapy on mortality of HIV-infected children.

	Adjusted* relative hazard (95% CI)
Therapy	
None	1.00 (reference)
Monotherapy	0.77 (0.55–1.08)
Double combination therapy	0.70 (0.42–1.17)
Triple combination therapy	0.29 (0.13–0.67)

* Relative hazards are adjusted for a number of variables including clinical stage, immunologic stage, receipt of pneumocystis pneumonia prophylaxis and stratified by clinical center.
Data from De Martino, M. *et al.* "Reduction in mortality with availability of antiretroviral therapy for children with perinatal HIV-1 infection." *JAMA* **284** (2000): 190–7.

9.2 What if I want to prove that an intervention is not inferior or is equivalent to another intervention?

> Superiority trials seek to prove that one treatment is better than another.

Up until this part of the book, we have been discussing how to determine whether persons in the intervention group do better (or worse) than subjects in the non-intervention group(s). This is called a superiority trial. However, sometimes the goal is to prove that one treatment is not inferior to another (a non-inferiority trial) or that two or more treatments are equivalent (an equivalence trial).[2]

The terms non-inferiority trial and equivalence trial are sometimes confused; although they have similarities, they are not the same. Because non-inferiority trials are much more common, I will review them first.

> Non-inferiority trials seek to demonstrate that a treatment is not substantially worse than another treatment.

Non-inferiority trials seek to demonstrate that a treatment is not substantially worse than another treatment. Non-inferiority trials are particularly important if one intervention is substantially less expensive, has fewer side effects, or has a higher rate of compliance than the standard intervention.

To perform a non-inferiority trial you must first define the size of the difference between the treatments that would lead you to conclude that a treatment is worse than the standard treatment. The amount should be the smallest difference between two treatments that would be clinically significant. In other words, if a new treatment were this much worse, you would stick with the standard treatment. The amount can be defined in percentages or points on a scale.

---

[2] For a particularly good paper on this topic see: Piaggio, G., Elbourne, D. R., Altman, D. G., *et al.* "Reporting of noninferiority and equivalence randomized trials: An extension of the CONSORT statement." *JAMA* **295** (2006): 1152–60. To go deeper into this complex field see: Kaul, S. and Diamond, G. A. "Good enough: A primer on the analysis and interpretation of noninferiority trials." *Ann. Intern. Med.* **145** (2006): 62–9; Gøtzsche, P. C. "Lessons from and cautions about noninferiority and equivalence randomized trials." *JAMA* **295** (2006): 1172–4. Djulbegovic, B. and Clarke, M. "Scientific and ethical issues in equivalence trials." *JAMA* **285** (2001): 1206–8.

Power calculations and statistical testing are based on the 95% confidence interval for the difference between the treatments being less than the preset threshold for what would be considered clinically worse.

For example, it is well known that continuous exercise benefits persons with chronic obstructive pulmonary disease. The problem is that continuous exercise can be difficult for persons with COPD, resulting in low compliance. Puhan and colleagues assessed whether interval exercise would have similar beneficial effects to continuous exercise.[3]

The investigators defined 45 meters in a 6-minute walking test as a clinically meaningful standard. In other words, if participants in the continuous intervention arm could walk 45 meters more than the participants in the interval intervention arm, then the interval intervention is inferior; if those in the continuous intervention arm cannot walk 45 meters more than those in the interval intervention arm, then interval exercise is not inferior.

Following the two interventions the adjusted difference between the two groups on the 6-minute walking test (distance walked by interval group – difference walked by continuous exercise group) was 1.1 meters. The 95% confidence interval was (–25.4 to 27.6). Because the confidence intervals did not include –45 meters the study demonstrated non-inferiority of interval exercise. Persons in the interval exercise group were more likely to adhere to the protocol (48% vs. 24%; $P = .0014$).

Two additional points about this study: I chose it because most people think of non-inferiority studies in the context of medication comparisons – I wanted to illustrate that the design can be used for non-medication trials. Second, the comparison of the two groups reported above was based on a per-protocol analysis, not an intention-to-treat analysis. From Section 4.8 you will remember my explaining that intention-to-treat analysis is preferred for randomized trials because it maintains the benefits of randomization. However, this is not necessarily the case for inferiority trials. The reason is that intention-to-treat analysis tends to bias towards the null finding, which would make it easier to demonstrate non-inferiority. That's why non-inferiority trials should use per-protocol analysis; ideally, per-protocol and intention-to-treat analyses will produce similar answers. (Although the main analysis reported by the investigators in this trial was the per-protocol analysis, they also reported the intention-to-treat analysis, which showed similar results.)

While non-inferiority studies seek to prove that the difference between the effect of an intervention is no worse than a preset standard, equivalence studies

> Non-inferiority trials should report the per-protocol analysis.

[3] Puhan, M. A., Busching, G., Schunemann, H. J., van Oort, E., Zaugg, C., and Frey, M. "Interval versus continuous high-intensity exercise in chronic obstructive pulmonary disease." *Ann. Intern. Med.* **145** (2006): 816–25.

> Equivalence studies seek to prove that two (or more) treatments are of similar value.

seek to prove that the difference between two (or more) interventions is no larger than a preset standard. In the language of statistical hypothesis testing, with non-inferiority studies we are only interested in one tail; with equivalence studies we are interested in two tails.

For example, Parienti *et al.* were interested in establishing that hand-rubbing with an aqueous alcohol solution and surgical hand-scrubbing were equivalent in terms of rates of surgical infections.[4] The investigators chose 2% as the difference in surgical infections that would be considered clinically relevant. Therefore, the power calculation for the study was based on assuming that the difference between the infection rates of the two treatments was 0 and the confidence intervals for that difference would be –2.0% to +2.0%. In other words, if the difference between the infection rates for the two groups was more than 2%, the treatments would not be equivalent.

Surgical infections occurred in 2.44% of the patients in the hand-rubbing group and 2.48% of the patients in the hand-washing group for a difference of 0.04% (95% CI = –0.88% to 0.96%). Because the 95% confidence intervals are well within the –2.0% to +2.0% boundary we can conclude that the two treatments are equal.

9.3 How do I adjust for multiple comparisons?

As discussed in Section 3.10, it is often advantageous to test whether an intervention affects more than one outcome. However, when performing multiple comparisons you may need to adjust for the number of comparisons you make.

The reason to consider adjusting for multiple comparisons is the concern that if we perform 20 comparisons between an intervention and a comparison, we would expect that one of the comparisons would be statistically significant at the $P = 0.05$ level by chance alone. Therefore, if one of 20 comparisons is significant, do we conclude that the intervention is effective for that outcome or do we conclude that we have a statistical artifact (this is the same issue with pairwise comparisons (Sections 6.2.A, 6.2.B and 6.4.B), subgroup analyses (Section 9.5), and interim analyses (Section 9.4))?

> If you are performing 2–4 comparisons, use the Bonferroni correction.

If you are performing only two to four comparisons, the simplest adjustment method is to use the Bonferroni correction just as you would do when making pairwise comparisons for an ANOVA design (Section 6.4.B). So if you were assessing the impact of the intervention on four outcomes you would divide

---

[4] Parienti, J. J., Thibon, P., and Heller, R., "Hand-rubbing with an aqueous alcoholic solution vs traditional surgical hand-scrubbing and 30-day surgical site infection rates: a randomized equivalence study." *JAMA* **288** (2002): 722–7.

the conventional P value of 0.05 by 4 and require that any comparison have a P value of less than 0.0125 (0.05/4) before concluding that the difference is statistically significant.

As with pairwise testing, the problem with the Bonferroni correction is that it is very conservative, especially when you have a large number of outcomes. For example, Morey and colleagues performed an intervention to improve functional outcomes among older, overweight cancer survivors.[5] The primary outcome of their study was a change in physical function. In addition they assessed 17 secondary outcomes. If they used the Bonferroni correction for their secondary outcomes the only comparisons that would be considered statistically significant would be those with P values less than 0.003 (0.5/17). Instead, as you can see in Table 9.3, they used an adaptation of the Bonferroni procedure, called the Holm procedure.

For the Holm procedure the P values for the different outcomes are ranked in sequential order from the lowest to the highest. The lowest P value has to be less than the Bonferroni threshold (in this case 0.003) to be statistically significant and to continue testing the remaining outcomes. As you continue assessing the outcomes in order, the denominator on the Bonferroni correction is decreased by one (0.003/16), (0.003/15), etc. This becomes the threshold against which you determine whether the comparison is statistically significant.

If you compare the final two columns you can see that in some cases a difference between the intervention group and the placebo group was below the 0.05 threshold, but did not reach statistical significance using the Holm test. For example, the difference between the groups on the advanced lower extremity function was not statistically significant using the more rigorous threshold.

> The major ambiguity with adjusting for multiple comparisons is the question of what comparisons to include.

For a variety of reasons, not everyone believes that adjustment for multiple comparisons is necessary.[6] A major reason is the ambiguity of what comparisons to count. For example, let's say you read the study by Morey and you were interested in whether the intervention improved sexual function of the elders (there is good evidence that exercise improves sexual function). You contact the investigators; they tell you that they did in fact collect data on sexual function and you are welcome to explore that question with their data (with appropriate attribution, of course). When you perform that comparison would you adjust your analysis for just the number of comparisons you were making (e.g., number of times a week for sex, satisfaction with sex, partner's satisfaction

[5] Morey, M. C., Snyder, D. C., Sloane, R., *et al.* "Effects of home-based diet and exercise on functional outcomes among older, overweight long-term cancer survivors." *JAMA* **301** (2009): 1883–91.

[6] Rothman, K. J. "No adjustments are needed for multiple comparisons." *Epidemiology* **1** (1990): 43–6.

Table 9.3. Differences between the intervention group and the control group on a primary outcome and 17 secondary outcomes.

	Mean (SE)		Mean group difference (95% CI)	Adjusted P value*	Holm procedure α level
	Intervention (n = 319) change at 12 mo	Control (n = 322) change at 12 mo			
Primary outcome					
SF-36 physical function (range, 0–100)	−2.15 (0.9)	−4.84 (0.9)	2.69 (0.17 to 5.21)	0.03	
Secondary outcomes					
LLF basic lower extremity function (range, 45.6–100)	0.34 (0.6)	−1.89 (0.6)	2.24 (0.56 to 3.91)	0.005	0.005
LLF advanced lower extremity function (range, 0–100)	−0.37 (0.5)	−2.30 (0.6)	1.92 (0.45 to 3.39)	0.02	0.006
Behavioral targets					
Duration of strength training exercise, min/wk (range, 0–600)	18.7 (2.4)	0.5 (2.7)	18.21 (11.21 to 25.21)	<0.001	0.003
Duration of endurance exercise, min/wk (range, 0–149)	36.3 (4.9)	23.4 (5.6)	12.89 (1.89 to 27.58)	0.004	0.004
Strength training exercise frequency, sessions/wk (range, 0–7)	1.4 (0.2)	0.2 (0.1)	1.12 (0.70 to 1.54)	<0.001	0.003
Endurance exercise frequency, sessions/wk (range, 0–15)	1.6 (0.2)	0.5 (0.2)	1.05 (0.39 to 1.72)	0.005	0.005
Daily servings of fruits and vegetables (range, 0–15.80)	1.24 (0.14)	0.13 (0.11)	1.11 (0.76 to 1.47)	<0.001	0.003
Sat. fat intake, g/d (range, 2–57 g)	−3.06 (0.51)	−1.07 (0.49)	−1.99 (−0.58 to −3.40)	0.002	0.004
Weight, kg (range, 59.1–125.5 kg)	−2.06 (0.19)	−0.92 (0.2)	−1.14 (−0.59 to −1.69)	<0.001	0.004
Body mass index (range, 25–47)	−0.69 (0.07)	−0.31 (0.08)	−0.38 (−0.19 to 0.57)	<0.001	0.004
Health-related quality of life on SF-36					
General health (range, 15–100)	0.77 (0.72)	−1.94 (0.80)	2.71 (0.58 to 4.84)	0.03	0.007
Pain (range, 10–100)	−0.78 (1.07)	−3.19 (1.22)	2.40 (−0.79 to 5.59)	0.16	0.02
Vitality (range, 0–100)	−0.47 (0.89)	−2.42 (0.98)	1.95 (−0.64 to 4.55)	0.10	0.01
Social functioning (range, 12.5–100)	−1.29 (1.05)	−5.05 (1.22)	3.75 (0.58 to 6.92)	0.03	0.008
Mental health (range, 32–100)	0.50 (0.53)	−2.04 (0.74)	2.54 (0.75 to 4.33)	0.01	0.006
Physical role (range, 0–100)	−2.43 (2.02)	−4.68 (2.14)	2.25 (−3.54 to 8.05)	0.32	0.03
Emotional role (range, 0–100)	−0.73 (1.32)	−0.62 (1.38)	−0.11 (−3.86 to 3.64)	0.93	0.05

* All models were adjusted for baseline value of the outcome, age, race, number of comorbidities, number of symptoms, education, cancer type, body mass index, and SF-36 physical function subscale score.

Data from Morey, M. C., Snyder, D. C., Sloane, R., *et al.* "Effects of home-based diet and exercise on functional outcomes among older, overweight long-term cancer survivors." *JAMA* **301** (2009): 1883–91.

with sex) or for the number of comparisons Morey and colleagues made in their paper plus the number you were making?

What if you identified 20 datasets that randomized persons to an exercise regimen and collected data on sexual function? Would you adjust for the number of comparisons you made using the 20 datasets? If you are thinking that it is far-fetched to adjust for comparisons in different datasets, consider this: if you were to compare the benefit of exercise in 20 different trials, you would expect that one of the trials would show benefit for exercise at the $P = 0.05$ threshold by chance alone. On the other hand, you wouldn't expect the 20 different investigators to adjust their data for the other 19 studies. In fact, they wouldn't even necessarily know the other studies were going on. It's a conundrum.

My general advice on this complicated topic is to:

1 Pre-specify the comparisons you intend to perform in your analysis plan (Section 3.11), including being clear what your primary outcome is (it is not necessary to adjust the primary analysis for the number of secondary comparisons).
2 Tell the reader how many comparisons have been made; that way even if you do not adjust for multiple comparisons, the reader can take the number of comparisons performed into account.
3 Don't be a slave to P values. Whether a comparison is just over or just under a threshold, whether that threshold is adjusted or not, is unlikely to be the major determinant of whether an intervention works. Other factors, including biological plausibility, consistency with other empiric findings, clinical effect size, elimination of confounding, success of blinding, drop out rates, intensity of exposure, contamination, missing data, dose–response relationship, are more likely determinants of whether the intervention really works.

9.4 Should a trial have pre-specified interim analyses with early stopping rules?

The purpose of interim analyses is to stop a trial early if there is sufficient evidence of effectiveness or harm.

When designing a trial you may want to plan for an interim data analysis. The purpose of interim analyses is to stop a trial early if there is sufficient difference between the groups to conclude that the intervention is effective or harmful. In the case of efficacy, early stopping may allow subjects in the placebo arm, and those not in the study at all, to receive the beneficial treatment sooner. In the case of side effects, early stopping may prevent unnecessary harm. Early stopping may also save money and facilitate earlier reporting and translation of the results to clinical practice.

The major problem with interim analysis is that by repeatedly "checking" to see whether there is a difference between the groups you are increasing the chance of making a type 1 error (falsely concluding that there is a difference between the groups when there is no difference). To appreciate why, imagine that you check whether there is a difference between your groups at 20 different times. We would expect, by chance alone, that the difference between the groups would be statistically significant at the $P = 0.05$ level at least once.

Therefore interim analyses set a more stringent P value to avoid prematurely concluding the study. These interim analyses are performed at pre-specified times – time is usually based on a percentage of study accrual (e.g., when 60% of the subjects have been enrolled in the study). At each pre-specified time the investigators will specify how large a difference between the two groups will constitute sufficient evidence to terminate the study.

The combination of pre-specified times for the early analysis and the threshold of the P value for ending the study early are referred to as early stopping rules. If there is more than one planned early analysis (e.g., when 50% of the subjects have been enrolled and when 70% of the subjects have been enrolled) the P value for ending at the first look will be more stringent than the P value for ending at a later time. The interim analysis should be performed by a data and safety monitoring committee (Section 3.14).

> Early stopping rules specify a time to test for differences and a P value needed to stop the study.

For example, Lallermant and colleagues planned interim analyses with early stopping rules for their trial of single-dose nevirapine plus zidovudine for the prevention of perinatal transmission of HIV.[7] The investigators enrolled 1844 women to one of three groups: (1) single-dose nevirapine for mother and infant (nevirapine–nevirapine regimen); (2) single-dose nevirapine for mother and placebo for infant (nevirapine–placebo regimen); (3) placebo for mother and infant (placebo–placebo). Patients and investigators were masked to treatment assignment (double-blinded).

The investigators planned to conduct the first interim analysis when 40% of the women were enrolled and a second interim analysis when 70% of the women were enrolled. An increase in the rate of HIV transmission associated with any of the three treatment regimens would be considered significant if any nominal P value was less than 0.0004 at the first interim analysis.

---

[7] Lallermant, M., Jourdain, G., Le Coeur, S., *et al.* "Single-dose perinatal nevirapine plus standard zidovudine to prevent mother-to-child transmission of HIV-1 in Thailand." *N. Engl. J. Med.* **351** (2004): 217–28.

Indeed, after reviewing the data at the first interim analysis, the independent data and safety monitoring committee recommended stopping enrollment in the placebo–placebo group. The transmission rate in women in the nevirapine–nevirapine group (1.1%, 95% confidence interval 0.3 to 2.2) was significantly lower than that in the placebo–placebo group (6.3%, 95% confidence interval 3.8 to 8.9%). No serious adverse reactions were reported with the single dose.

I chose this example because the stakes of this study were so high (preventing HIV infection) that you can really appreciate the benefits of early stopping rules. We wouldn't want to continue giving women placebo if we have enough information to say that infection rates are lower with treatment and the treatment is safe.

However, early stopping rules may not always be a good idea. Montori and colleagues conducted a systemic review of randomized controlled trials that were stopped early because of greater benefit in one group.[8] They found that many studies did not report the planned sample size for interim analysis, or whether a stopping rule informed the decision, or whether the interim analysis was adjusted for interim monitoring. Although these are problems that can be fixed, they also found that many trials that were stopped with few events yielded implausibly large treatment effects, suggesting that they may have caught a random high.

> Interim analyses may hit a random high or low.

The chance of catching a random high (or low) can be made smaller by using more stringent cut-offs for early termination; on the other hand, more stringent cut-offs may make it impossible for a study to be terminated earlier, in which case there is no purpose to an interim analysis.

There are two other issues of interest concerning interim analyses. The data and safety subcommittee members need not unblind the study to perform an interim analysis. They can simply compare the groups on the pre-specified criteria. If there is a sufficiently large difference between the groups that the study will be terminated early, the subcommittee members can then unblind the data and determine which group was doing better.

When you have a well-publicized study that is known to have interim analyses, researchers and clinicians in the field will draw conclusions when the interim analysis is conducted and no study termination occurs. They will assume that the treatment difference is not large. However, just as there can be random highs, there can be random lows, and a drug may turn out to be effective when a sufficient number of events have occurred.

---

[8] Montori, V. M., Devereaux, P. J., Adhikari, N. K. J., *et al.* "Randomized trials stopped early for benefit." *JAMA* **294** (2005): 2203–9.

9.5 How do I analyze subgroup differences in the response to an intervention?

<table>
<tr>
<td>

Subgroups may be defined by baseline characteristics, comorbid conditions, or severity of illness.

</td>
</tr>
</table>

It is often of interest to know whether an intervention works better (or worse) for different groups. The subgroups are typically defined by baseline characteristics such as demographics (e.g., does aspirin have a greater benefit among men than women in preventing heart disease?), presence of comorbid conditions (e.g., do ACE inhibitors have greater benefit among diabetics than non-diabetics?) and severity of disease (e.g., do HIV antiretroviral drugs have greater benefit in patients with severe immunodeficiency than patients with normal immune function?).

<table>
<tr>
<td>

Subgroup analysis has a bad reputation!

</td>
</tr>
</table>

Given the obvious importance of subgroup analysis it may seem surprising that it has such a bad reputation. Why? The reason is that some investigators have mistakenly claimed to find an effect in subgroup analyses when all they really found was statistical artifact. Here's how.

Let's imagine that you compare an intervention to placebo in 200 people. You find that the intervention has no effect compared to placebo. You then compare the intervention to placebo in men and women separately. No difference. You then compare the intervention to placebo across ethnicities. No difference in any ethnic group. You then compare the intervention to placebo among the young and the old. You find that the intervention is significantly better for the old but not the young. You are excited to have finally identified a significant value and draft a manuscript on how the intervention works for older people. Wrong! Why?

<table>
<tr>
<td>

If you compare an intervention to placebo in enough different subgroups you would expect that the intervention would differ from placebo in at least one of the groups by chance alone.

</td>
</tr>
</table>

If you compare an intervention to placebo in enough different subgroups you would expect that the intervention would differ from placebo in at least one of the groups by chance alone. Note this is the same reason that when performing multiple interim analyses (Section 9.4) you need to pre-specify when you will be performing the analysis and you must use a more stringent P value to determine statistical significance.

<table>
<tr>
<td>

Use interaction terms to demonstrate subgroup differences.

</td>
</tr>
</table>

Another reason subgroup analysis has a bad reputation is that investigators make a common statistical mistake in analyzing this type of data: concluding that there is a difference between groups based on separate analyses of each group (e.g., determining the odds ratio for the intervention versus placebo among men and separately determining the odds ratio for the intervention versus placebo among women).[9] To demonstrate that there is a statistically significant difference across subgroups you must demonstrate that there is a statistically significant interaction term.

[9] Wang, R., Lagakos, S. W., Ware, J. H., Hunter, D. J., and Drazen, J. M. "Statistics in medicine – reporting of subgroup analyses in clinical trials." *N. Engl. J. Med.* **357** (2007): 2189–94.

Table 9.4. Illustration that the components of an interaction term plus the interaction term define four unique groups.

	Intervention, male sex	Intervention, female sex	Non-intervention, male sex	Non-intervention, female sex
Intervention vs. no intervention	1	1	0	0
Male vs. female	1	0	1	0
Interaction term (intervention × male sex)	1	0	0	0

To construct an interaction term multiply the intervention term by the subgroup. If the intervention variable is (1 = yes; 0 = no) and the subgroup is male sex (1 = yes; 0 = no), then the interaction term will take on two values (0 or 1); the group with both characteristics will be the only group with a value of one as shown below:

Intervention group and male sex = 1 x 1 = **1**
Intervention group and female sex = 1 x 0 = **0**
Non-intervention group and male sex = 0 x 1 = **0**
Non-intervention group and female sex = 0 x 0 = **0**

Although the only group with a value of one is the first group, you can see from the columns of Table 9.4 that the three variables (shown in the rows) – the intervention term, the sex term, and the interaction term – define four unique groups.

Let's assume that the outcome of this hypothetical study is rupture of an aortic aneurysm. If the intervention is effective in reducing ruptures then the variable intervention (row 1) will be statistically significant. If males have more ruptures than females the variable male sex will be statistically significant (row 2). If the intervention is statistically more or less effective among men than women, the interaction term (row 3) will be statistically significant.

Armed with the knowledge of how to test whether an interaction is statistically significant, there are two correct ways of performing subgroup analyses: with a pre-specified analysis plan (Section 3.11) or with tremendous humility.

> There are two correct ways of performing subgroup analyses: with a pre-specified analysis plan or with tremendous humility.

At the outset of a study there may be reason to suspect that an intervention will work better in one group than another. Go ahead and describe in the analysis plan your intention to study whether the intervention works equally well in both groups. Power your analysis sufficiently for this comparison. If you are performing a randomized trial, you may wish to use a stratified allocation of subjects (Section 4.4) to be sure you have a sufficient number of subjects in each group.

Even if you don't identify subgroup analysis as part of a pre-specified plan, you may discover in conducting your study, or in analyzing your data, that there are differences across subgroups. It is fine to go ahead and explore those differences, but this is post-hoc analysis (Section 3.11). Show tremendous humility in reporting the results.

9.6 How should I deal with missing data in my intervention study?

Handling missing data is a challenge in any kind of study. With intervention studies, it is common to have missing data on baseline characteristics (covariates), especially if the subjects were drawn from medical records, registries, or administrative databases.

> The easiest method for dealing with missing data is to delete cases with missing values on important covariates.

If you have a very small number of cases with missing data on covariates, it is easiest to simply delete those cases from your analysis. If the number of deleted cases is a small proportion of your total sample (e.g., < 3%), and the cases with missing data are not different from cases without missing data on other prognostic factors, deleting them is unlikely to bias your analysis.

> If you have a large number of missing values on certain variables it may be better to delete the variables from the analysis rather than the cases.

At the other extreme, if you have variables with a large number of missing cases (e.g., > 15%), the best solution may be to delete these variables (rather than the cases) from the analysis. No matter how important the variables may be to your theory, if you have a lot of missing cases on these variables, including them in the analysis will lead to loss of cases (if you exclude cases with missing data) or potential measurement error (if you must estimate the missing values using multiple imputation: see below.)

> Multiple imputation is the best way to incorporate subjects with missing values on covariates.

When the number of cases you would lose by excluding those with missing values is not trivial and when your covariates have some (but not a substantial proportion) of missing values the best way to incorporate these cases is to use multiple imputation to estimate the missing values.[10] Multiple imputation is a sophisticated method of estimating the value of missing values, based on the values of those subjects with complete data on the missing variable and its important correlates. In addition a random component with repetition is used to compute standard errors that take into account the uncertainty induced by imputing the value.

With a longitudinal study, where the outcome is measured repeatedly, there may also be missing outcome data (e.g., a subject attends the first five study appointments but misses the sixth one). In situations such as these, many analytic methods (e.g., ANOVA, conditional logistic regression) cannot be used because they require the same number of observations per subject.

---

[10] For more on multiple imputation see: Heitjan, D. F. "What can be done about missing data? Approaches to imputation." *Am. J. Public Health* **87** (1997): 548–50; Rubin, D. B. *Multiple Imputation for Nonresponse in Surveys.* New York: Wiley, 1987. For a more general discussion of how to handle missing data including multiple imputation see Katz, M. H. *Multivariable Analysis: A Practical Guide for Clinicians.* Cambridge: Cambridge University Press, 2006: pp. 87–94.

In cases where there is a very small percentage of subjects with a missing observation, and these subjects are no different from those subjects with all their values, it is possible to exclude these subjects from your analysis. Unfortunately this results in loss of sample size.

> Don't carry the last observation forward to deal with missing data.

In the past it was common to deal with this problem by carrying the last observation forward. With this method the missing value is replaced with the most recent valid non-missing value. Unfortunately, this method can result in underestimating or overestimating the treatment effect and should not be used.[11]

A better method of dealing with missing observations is to use an analytic method that can incorporate missing observations such as generalized estimating equations and mixed-effects models. Both can deal with data that are missing randomly and may be able to deal with nonrandomly missing data when the outcome is interval (but not dichotomous).[12]

9.7 What special considerations are there for publishing the results of intervention trials?

A major improvement in the field of intervention research has been the establishment of guidelines for publishing studies. The guidelines ensure that investigators include all relevant information in their manuscripts. By standardizing the presentation of results, guidelines also help readers to rapidly find the information they are looking for and make it easier to compare the results of trials, informally and through meta-analysis. There is a guideline for publishing randomized intervention trials[13] and an extension of this guideline for non-inferiority and equivalence randomized trials.[14] For publishing nonrandomized studies, two guidelines are available.[15]

---

[11] Streiner, D. L. "The case of the missing data: Methods of dealing with dropouts and other research vagaries." *Can. J. Psychiatry* **47** (2002): 68–75; Molnar, F. J., Hutton, B., and Fergusson, D. "Does analysis using 'last observation carried forward' introduce bias in dementia research?" *CMAJ* **179** (2008). www.cmaj.ca/cgi/content/full/179/8/751

[12] For a general discussion of inclusion of missing data in generalized estimating equations and mixed effects models see: Katz, M. H. *Multivariable Analysis: A Practical Guide for Clinicians.* Cambridge: Cambridge University Press, 2006: pp. 164–71.

[13] Moher, D., Shulz, K. F., and Altman, D., for the CONSORT group. "The CONSORT statement: Revised recommendations for improving the quality of reports of parallel-group randomized trials." *JAMA* **285** (2001): 1887–91.

[14] Piaggio, G., Elbourne, D. R., Altman, D. G., Pocock, S. J., and Evans S. J. W., for the CONSORT Group. "Reporting of noninferiority and equivalence randomized trials: An extension of the CONSORT statement." *JAMA* **295** (2006): 1152–60.

[15] Des Jarlais, D. C., Lyles, C., Crepaz, N., and the TREND Group. "Improving the reporting quality of nonrandomized evaluations of behavioral and public health interventions: The Trend statement." *Am. J. Public Health* **94** (2004): 361–6; Von Elm, E., Altman, D. G., Egger, M., *et al.* "The strengthening of the reporting of observational studies in epidemiology (STROBE) statement: Guidelines for reporting observational studies." *J. Clin. Epidemiol.* **61** (2008): 344–9.

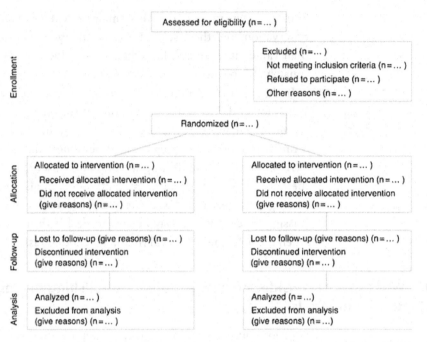

Figure 9.2   Flow diagram for trial. Reprinted with permission from Moher, D., *et al.* ``The CONSORT statement: revised recommendations for improving the quality of reports of parallel-group randomized trials. *JAMA*. 2001, **285**: 1987–91. Copyright © (2001) American Medical Association. All rights reserved.

> All trials should have a Figure 1 showing the flow of subjects through the study.

The guidelines themselves are very detailed, and I won't attempt to review them in full. But I do want to stress the importance of including a diagram showing the flow of subjects through a trial. A generic version of such a figure is shown in Figure 9.2.[16]

Figure 9.3 is from a study of physical activity on cognitive function in patients at risk for Alzheimer disease.[17] Starting at the top of the figure and working your way down, note how the figure enables you to quickly assess who is excluded and why.

Continuing down from the branch point it is easy to see how many subjects were randomized into each group, and within each group, and how many subjects completed the 6-month, 12-month, and 18-month assessments, along

---

[16] Moher, D., Schulz, K. F., Altman, D., for the CONSORT Group. "The CONSORT statement: revised recommendations for improving the quality of reports of parallel group trials. *JAMA* (2001) **285**: 1987–91.

[17] Lautenschlager, N. T., Cox, K. L., Flicker, *et al.* "Effect of physical activity or cognitive function in older adults at risk for Alzheimer disease." *JAMA* **300** (2008): 1027–37.

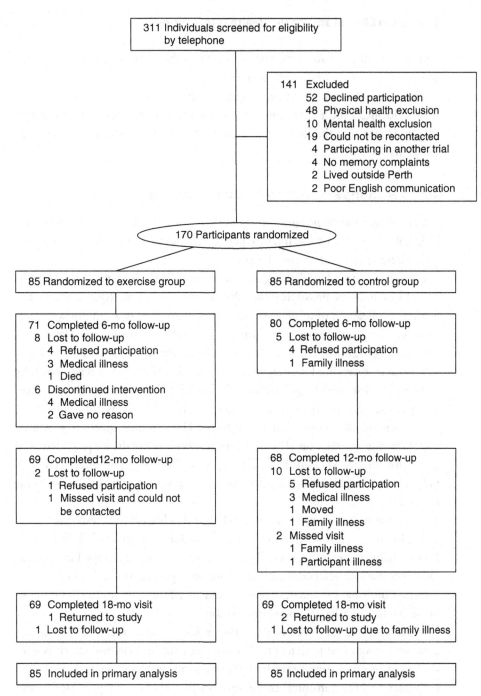

311 Individuals screened for eligibility
by telephone

141 Excluded
52 Declined participation
48 Physical health exclusion
10 Mental health exclusion
19 Could not be recontacted
4 Participating in another trial
4 No memory complaints
2 Lived outside Perth
2 Poor English communication

170 Participants randomized

85 Randomized to exercise group

85 Randomized to control group

71 Completed 6-mo follow-up
8 Lost to follow-up
4 Refused participation
3 Medical illness
1 Died
6 Discontinued intervention
4 Medical illness
2 Gave no reason

80 Completed 6-mo follow-up
5 Lost to follow-up
4 Refused participation
1 Family illness

69 Completed 12-mo follow-up
2 Lost to follow-up
1 Refused participation
1 Missed visit and could not
be contacted

68 Completed 12-mo follow-up
10 Lost to follow-up
5 Refused participation
3 Medical illness
1 Moved
1 Family illness
2 Missed visit
1 Family illness
1 Participant illness

69 Completed 18-mo visit
1 Returned to study
1 Lost to follow-up

69 Completed 18-mo visit
2 Returned to study
1 Lost to follow-up due to family illness

85 Included in primary analysis

85 Included in primary analysis

Figure 9.3   Flow diagram for randomized study of the impact of physical activity on cognitive function in patients at risk for Alzheimer's disease. Reprinted with permission from Lautenschlager, N. T., *et al.* "Effect of physical activity on cognitive function in older adults at risk for Alzheimer disease." *JAMA* **300** (2008): 1027–37. © 2008 American Medical Association. All rights reserved.

with the number of subjects who were lost to follow-up or discontinued the intervention at each of these time points.

The very bottom of the flow diagram indicates that the primary analysis was performed on the same number of subjects as were initially randomized. This indicates that the investigators conducted an intention-to-treat analysis (Sections 3.9, 5.8).

9.8 What special considerations are there for publishing negative studies?

Studies where the intervention does not work are less likely to get published (Section 3.9) or at least less likely to get published in the most prestigious journals. There are several reasons for this.

One reason for not publishing a negative study is that it isn't sufficiently powerful to exclude the possibility that the intervention works (type 2 error). For example, colleagues of mine were interested in answering an important question: how to get more persons at high risk of HIV to enroll in available HIV prevention programs. Our earlier work had shown that less than 6% of high-risk patients receiving HIV-negative test results at the San Francisco sexually transmitted disease (STD) clinic had received an HIV-prevention referral; how many of the 6% actually followed through on the referral was not known.[18]

To increase the proportion of high-risk HIV-negative persons receiving and following through on HIV-prevention service referrals, we provided HIV counselors at the STD clinic with training on how to more effectively provide referrals to patients; counselors were also given detailed lists of available referrals.[19]

Since counselors at the STD clinic believed that high-risk HIV-negative persons did not perceive themselves to be at risk for HIV and had little motivation to follow through on referrals, an intervention was developed to increase follow-through on referrals by having counselors give clients additional referral information, ongoing encouragement and assistance, reminders, and reimbursements for childcare and transportation.

Clients were randomized to the intervention or to usual care. A power calculation showed that to detect a 10% improvement in accessing referrals with the intervention (assuming the intervention group accessed referrals with 20% frequency and the non-intervention group with 10% frequency), a sample size

[18] Marx, R., Hirozawa, A. M., Chu, P. L., Bolan, G. A., and Katz, M. H. "Linking clients from HIV antibody counseling and testing to prevention services." *J. Community Health* **24** (1999): 201–13.
[19] Marx, R., Sebesta, D. S., Hirozawa, A. M., *et al.*, "Can follow-through on HIV prevention referrals be increased among high-risk seronegative individuals? An exploratory study"; unpublished paper.

of 200 per group would be needed (assumes power of 80% and two-sided statistical testing at alpha = 0.05).

Given the high volume of high-risk patients coming to the STD clinic it should have been possible to recruit a sample of this size, but for a variety of reasons it wasn't. Over a 14-month period, only 113 of the 121 persons who met study criteria agreed to participate, and only 79 were available for baseline interviews. Of these 79 clients, 39 were randomized to the intervention and 40 to the non-intervention group. However, the effective sample size was even smaller than this because the intervention could only be done for patients who did not access referrals prior to the intervention and who were available for a follow-up interview. In this small group, there was no difference in follow-up of referrals between the two groups: only 2 of 16 intervention clients (12.5%) versus 2 of 22 non-intervention clients (9.1%) ($P = 1.0$).

The 95% confidence interval for the odds ratio of 1.4 was 0.18 to 11.38. In other words, the investigators could not rule out that the intervention could substantially increase or decrease follow-through on prevention referrals. For this reason, the data really could not inform next steps and were not published.

However, even if you power your study such that you can rule out that the intervention works, you may still find it hard to publish? Why? Because there remains a bias against negative studies among journal reviewers and editors. This is unfortunate. A well done study that is adequately powered and evaluates an intervention that is either in use or may be potentially useful deserves the same attention whether the intervention works or not. Favoring studies with positive results encourages investigators to slant their results to demonstrate effects when the results are equivocal. If you've done a good study, don't be any less proud of it just because the intervention didn't work.

> Be proud of well done negative studies.

Research to action

10.1 How do you translate research into practice?

Many highly skilled researchers – able to develop, implement, and evaluate cutting-edge interventions – often fall short on the last, and most important, stage of the process: translating their research into practice.

Much of the problem is that the people who develop and evaluate interventions are usually academics, and academia is primarily concerned with generating new knowledge. Translating interventions into the messy world of government bureaucracies, public health departments, and social service agencies, as well as dealing with political and funding challenges, has never been the focus of academic work.

With medication and medical devices there exists a machinery – drug companies and medical device suppliers – to translate research findings into practice, including convincing doctors to prescribe them, patients to take them, and insurance companies to pay for them. No comparable machinery exists for behavioral or structural interventions (e.g., changes to the physical environment, changes to the law). Political leaders, public health and social service practitioners and advocates do not typically read research journals, and when they do they are often unsure how to translate projects that were conducted in a research setting into practice.

This gap between knowledge generation and program adoption must be bridged if we are to take full advantage of newly developed interventions. There are a number of steps that researchers can take to make translation of their work easier:

- Design interventions that are translatable.
- Articulate the benefits of the intervention in terms people will understand and be motivated by.
- Use the media to disseminate the results.
- Gain the support of interest groups.
- Send the results to policy makers.
- Develop a tool kit to make it easier to adopt the intervention.

Design interventions that are translatable.

　　In Section 2.2.C, I discussed the importance of developing interventions that are likely to be implemented. Interventions that have been shown to be effective, especially in real-world settings, are inexpensive, do not require highly specialized equipment or staff, and are of interest to the target population, are the ones most likely to be implemented.

Articulate the benefits of the intervention in terms people will understand and be motivated by.

　　For people to be interested in your intervention you will need to clearly articulate its benefits. Will people feel better? Will they save money? Will they live longer? If the intervention is aimed at physicians, will the intervention help them to practice better? Will it save them time? Will their patients feel better?

　　If you are aiming to convince politicians of the need to implement a law, they will want to know what advantage the law will provide for their constituents. Will it improve their services? Will it save them money?

　　Often local leaders can be persuaded to adopt a policy if it is considered to be a "best practice" in other parts of the world. For example, when I was convincing local politicians to have San Francisco become the first city in the United States to ban the sales of tobacco in pharmacies, I emphasized that a similar ban had been passed 10 years earlier in Canadian provinces.[1] This made it seem like a less radical idea.

Use the media to disseminate your results.

　　Many researchers are frightened by the press, thinking that reporters will try to sensationalize their results. Although it is true that the job of journalists is to sell newspapers (or magazines, TV advertisement time, web ads, etc.), journalists do not like to get the facts wrong. When stories are wrong it is often because no one took the time to explain to the reporter the findings in an understandable way.

　　To promote your findings, prepare a press release with a focus on what is new and exciting about your findings (detailing how your study confirms the results of prior studies is not likely to get much play). Send it out to newspapers and media outlets that will be interested. Give them lists of people to talk to, with phone numbers and emails, especially people not directly involved in the study who can attest to the broader implications of the work; follow up with phone conversations to the reporters.

Gain the support of interest groups.

　　Individuals do not change the world. Groups of individuals change the world. The best way to get the attention of policy makers is to line up several advocacy groups who support the intervention. For example, the American Heart Association and the American Lung Association were critical in pushing through smoking bans in the United States.

　　Who are the natural supporters of your intervention? Get them involved in advocating for it.

---

[1] Katz, M. H. "Banning tobacco sales in pharmacies: The right prescription." *JAMA* **300** (2008): 1451–3.

Engage policy makers.

As someone who works within a government bureaucracy, I chuckle when I read scholarly articles that include recommendations to policy makers. Few policy makers I know read scholarly articles. To engage policy makers, make an appointment with them and bring them copies of the research, but also "one-pagers" explaining the intervention and its value in easy-to-understand language. Tell them who supports your intervention and why. Also tell them who opposes it (policy makers hate being surprised by a group of angry constituents) and how their opposition can be neutralized.

Develop a tool kit to make it easier to adopt your work.

Interventions take time to implement. To increase implementation of an intervention create a tool kit. A tool kit should include background on the problem that the intervention is meant to address, descriptions of how to conduct the intervention, and the materials necessary to accomplish the goal. For example, when my county created a universal health coverage program,[2] we received many inquiries from other counties interested in pursuing similar initiatives. To make it as easy as possible, we asked a health foundation to create a tool kit for our program that included descriptions of the program, authorizing legislation, financing plan, quarterly charges, and point-of-service costs.

10.2 How is the translation of interventions assessed?

Use the RE-AIM (reach, efficacy/effectiveness, adoption, implementation, maintenance) framework to assess the translation of interventions.

A framework has been developed for assessing the translation of public health interventions, called RE-AIM.[3] Although the success of translating an intervention can usually be judged in less formal ways, the framework is helpful in assessing the different stages of implementation.

RE-AIM stands for reach, efficacy or effectiveness, adoption, implementation, and maintenance. Reach refers to the proportion of the target population who participated in the program and the characteristics of those persons. Participant characteristics are important to ensure that the program is reaching those who most need it (e.g., implementing an exercise program that attracts only persons who are already fit will not change obesity levels in the community).

Efficacy/effectiveness refers to the success rate when implemented as recommended. Adoption refers to the proportion of settings (e.g., clinics, community centers) that adopt the intervention. Implementation is the extent to which the program is implemented as recommended. Maintenance is the extent to which the program is sustained over time.

---

[2] Katz, M. H. "Golden Gate to health care for all? San Francisco's new universal-access program." *N. Engl. J. Med.* **358** (2008): 327–9.

[3] Glasgow, R. E., Vogt, T. M., and Boles, S. M. "Evaluating the public health impact of health promotion interventions: the RE-AIM framework." *Am. J. Public Health* **89** (1999): 1322–7.

For example, Li and colleagues used the RE-AIM framework to assess the translation of a tai chi intervention to six community senior centers in five cities in Oregon, USA.[4] In terms of reach, of the 555 persons who usually attend activities at the six community centers from which participants were enrolled, 287 signed up for the class and 249 were eligible to participate (reach = 249/555 or 45%). Participants were similar to the general population of senior center users.

In terms of effectiveness, participants showed significant pre-intervention to post-intervention improvement (Section 6.2) on a variety of physical measures. Adoption of the intervention by the six centers was 100% and all centers successfully implemented the program (implementation = 100%). Maintenance of the program was high (five centers continued offering the implementation beyond the study period and one was waiting for instructor availability).

[4] Li, R., Harmer, P., and Glasgow, R., *et al.* "Translation of an effective Tai Chi intervention into a community-based falls-prevention program." *Am. J. Public Health* **98** (2008): 1195–8.

11

Conclusion

Studying interventions is hard work, especially when the interventions do not lend themselves to randomized controlled designs! This is one reason that risk-factor studies greatly outnumber intervention studies in many critical areas, such as disparities in health outcomes, HIV transmission, substance abuse, and violence.

But the pay-off of developing, studying, and translating interventions into practice – changing the world – is tremendous. Early in my career, I published many descriptive and risk-factor studies. They helped me hone my statistical skills and some may have been of help to others in designing interventions. But I am proudest of the work that I have done developing and implementing interventions, so much so that I no longer perform risk-factor studies (although I still help people with theirs, while trying to recruit them to do intervention studies). I hope that this book will recruit you to the world of intervention studies.

If you need help (or you want to tell me about your success developing, evaluating, or implementing interventions) email me at mhkatz59@yahoo.com.

Index

Printed in the United States
By Bookmasters